SOMATIC EXERCISES for TRAUMA AND ANXIETY [2 in 1]:

40+ Illustrated Somatic Exercises & 30+ guided worksheets to relieve stress, anxiety, and recover from Past Trauma through Body-Mind Connection for beginners

Dr. Somatree Bells

Copyright © Dr. Somatree Bells

All rights reserved. No part of this book may be reproduced in any form without permission in writing from the publisher except in the case of brief quotations embodied in critical articles or reviews.

Legal & Disclaimer

The information contained in this book and its contents is not designed to replace or take the place of any form of medical or professional advice; and is not meant to replace the need for independent medical, financial, legal or other professional advice or services, as may be required. The content and information in this book have been provided for educational and entertainment purposes only.

Upon using the contents and information contained in this book, you agree to hold harmless the Author from and against any damages, costs, and expenses, including any legal fees potentially resulting from the application of any of the information provided by this book. This disclaimer applies to any loss, damages or injury caused by the use and application, whether directly or indirectly, of any advice or information presented, whether for breach of contract, tort, negligence, personal injury, criminal intent, or under any other cause of action.

You agree to accept all risks of using the information presented inside this book. By continuing to read this book, where appropriate and/or necessary, you shall consult a professional (including but not limited to your doctor, attorney, or financial advisor or such other advisor as needed) before using any of the suggested remedies, techniques, or information in this book.

Table of Contents

INTRODUCTION	**5**
WHAT IS SOMATIC EXERCISE?	**9**
WHY DO WE DO SOMATIC EXERCISES?	**11**
How Do We Do Somatic Exercise?	16
How Does Somatic Exercise Affect Trauma?	18
Nutrition and trauma recovery	19
How Diet Affects Mood and Anxiety	20
TRAUMA RECOVERY EXERCISES	**25**
40+ SOMATIC EXERCISES WITH DETAILED AND BASIC INSTRUCTIONS	**28**
LONG-TERM STRATEGIES FOR SUSTAINED HEALING	**67**
GROUP THERAPY AND COMPONENTS	**74**
A PATHWAY TO EASING ANXIETY THROUGH SOMATIC THERAPY	**77**
WORKSHEET FOR SOMATIC THERAPY AND ANXIETY	**81**
Exercise 1:	81
Exercise 2:	87
Exercise 3:	94
SOMATIC THERAPY WORKBOOK	**98**
SECTION 1: PREPARATION	**99**
Part 1: Body Awareness Scan	99
Part 2: Grounding Techniques	113
Part 3: Breathe Awareness	127
SECTION 2: EXPLORATION	**139**
Part 1: Body Mapping and Tracking	139
Part 2: Emotional Release Techniques	156
Part 3: Exploring Trauma Timeline	164
SECTION 3: HEALING TOOLS	**178**
Part 1: Self Holding and Compassion	178

PART 2: PROGRESSIVE MUSCLE RELAXATION	186
PART 3: SOMATIC YOGA SEQUENCES	197
SECTION 4: INTEGRATION	**200**
PART 1: DAILY ROUTINE	200
PART 2: REFLECTIVE JOURNALING	212
28-DAY EXERCISE PLAN	**220**
THE TRAUMA-HEALING DIET	**223**
CONCLUSION	**228**
CLAIM YOUR BONUSES HERE	**231**
REFERENCES	**233**

Introduction

I remember sitting across from Mel, her hands clasped tightly in her lap, her eyes darting around the consulting room. She had been to countless therapists and tried every medication under the sun, but the panic attacks still gripped her; the nightmares still haunted her sleep.

She looked at me with hope and desperation, "I don't know what else to do."

Her words echoed my own silent plea from years ago. I, too, had walked this path where the shadow of my past trauma looms large. But unlike Mel, I had stumbled upon a path less travelled: **somatic therapy.**

Somatic therapy isn't about talking your way out of trauma; it's about feeling your way through it. It's about reconnecting with your body, the silent keeper of your pain, and learning to listen to it. It was through this body-mind connection that I finally found relief, a way to soothe my troubled heart, calm my restless mind, and gently release my inner peace from the pole of trauma that had held me captive for so long.

I shared my experience with Mel, the simple yet powerful exercises that helped me ground myself in the present moment, release trapped emotions, and cultivate a sense of safety within my own skin.

As she started to incorporate these practices into her life, I saw a spark ignite within her. She now became much more alive. Her shoulders softened, her breath deepened, and a flicker of hope returned to her eyes.

This didn't only happen to Mel, but countless others who I share my tips and wellness ideas with through my newsletter. So, ***"Somatic Therapy for Trauma and anxiety"*** is me bringing my recovery and other people's recovery to more people. This is for them to discover the transformative power of somatic healing, to experience the freedom and joy of reclaiming their body and mind.

That's how this book came to be. It's a culmination of my personal journey, the lessons I've learned from my clients, and the wisdom gleaned from years of study and practice. It's a **guidebook**, **a workbook**, and **a companion**, all rolled into one.

Now to trauma: It is an emotional response to events such as rape, accidents, and other natural disasters. These events manifest as stressful, frightening, and distressing situations that are challenging to cope with and often beyond our control. Traumatic experiences can be singular incidents or ongoing events that occur over an extended period.

Many of us will encounter experiences that could be categorized as traumatic at some point in our lives, and you may have already experienced such events yourself. However, not everyone responds to trauma in the same manner. And because there are no age barriers to trauma, it can impact individuals at any stage of life. Sometimes, it surfaces long after the triggering event has occurred.

When these traumatic events happen, feelings of shock and denial are common reactions that follow. This could result to a range of longer-term effects over time including unpredictable emotions, flashbacks, strained relationships, and physical symptoms such as nausea and headaches. While these reactions are normal and prevalent for some people, many individuals struggle to move forward and resume their normal lives following a traumatic experience.

This book, *"Somatic Exercises for Trauma and Anxiety,"* aims to provide readers with practical exercises, answers and techniques designed to help manage and alleviate the symptoms of trauma and anxiety. By engaging with the somatic exercises outlined in this book, you will be able to reconnect with your body, regulate your emotions, and experience healing and resilience in the face of trauma or what makes you overly anxious.

This book will expose you to various somatic exercises that address different aspects of trauma and anxiety, offering a holistic approach to healing that encompasses the mind, body, and spirit.

In these pages, you'll find over **40 illustrated somatic exercises**, carefully curated to help you relieve stress, ease anxiety, and gently process past traumas. You'll find **30 guided worksheets** designed to help you explore your emotions, connect with your body, and rewrite your story.

Whether you are a trauma survivor seeking self-help tools or a healthcare professional looking to expand your therapeutic skills, this book offers valuable insights and strategies for promoting healing and recovery.

Also, it doesn't matter whether you're a beginner or have some experience with somatic practices, this book is for you. It's a safe space to explore, experiment, and find what works best for you.

Remember, healing is not a race; it's a journey. And that's why **the additional resources** in this book will help you to keep going even when you're done with the exercises from this workbook.

Take your time, be patient with yourself, and most importantly, listen to your body through the exercises in this book.

What is Somatic Exercise?

Somatic exercises involve the intricate connection between the mind and body, serving as a pathway to introspection and understanding of one's internal self. It encourages individuals to tune into the signals their bodies are sending, whether related to pain, imbalance, or discomfort. Somatic therapy utilizes this mind-body connection as a foundational approach to mental health treatment.

For those acquainted with alternative wellness practices, the term "somatics" may sound familiar, yet its precise meaning may remain difficult to catch. Somatic exercises offer a unique opportunity to gain insights into the ways in which experiences are stored and manifested within the body. This practice emphasizes presence and awareness during movement, fostering a deeper connection with one's body. Somatic experts believe that combining this awareness with natural movement and touch can significantly contribute to an individual's journey towards healing and overall wellness.

Engaging in somatic exercises involves cultivating a genuine connection with your body and attuning to its internal needs, rather than focusing solely on external goals or outcomes. This practice encourages mindfulness of the muscles being engaged, awareness of areas of tension within the body, and responsiveness to the body's signals. By doing so, you can access somatic energy, allowing your internal needs to guide you in a manner that alleviates tension and enhances genuine well-being.

The practice of somatic exercise has gained recognition over time for its effectiveness in relieving chronic pain by enhancing body awareness and promoting self-management of symptoms. Additionally, it helps to address trauma stored within the body, a phenomenon that many people may be unaware of.

The body has a remarkable ability to retain unresolved emotions and experiences, often manifesting as physical tension or discomfort. For instance, many women experience tight hips as a result of stored emotions, highlighting the profound impact of emotional experiences on physical well-being.

Renowned trauma expert, Dr. Bessel van der Kolk, has emphasized that trauma can literally reshape the body, underscoring the interconnectedness of emotional experiences and physical health. Even if you do not experience chronic pain or believe you have stored emotional tension, somatic exercise can still offer numerous benefits. From improving posture and addressing tight pelvic floor muscles to enhancing muscular strength, somatic exercises enable individuals to cultivate new, healthier muscular habits and promote overall wellness.

Why Do We Do Somatic Exercises?

Somatic exercises are a powerful way to improve your overall health, helping both your body and mind. Scientific research supports the efficacy of somatic movement in alleviating chronic pain, enhancing flexibility, balance, and mobility, and promoting emotional well-being.

Research studies have demonstrated that individuals experiencing chronic pain who engage in regular somatic exercises can achieve significant reductions in pain frequency and intensity. For instance, a study revealed that individuals who participated in somatic exercises for a year experienced an eighty-six percent reduction in the number of days they experienced pain compared to those who did not engage in somatic exercises.

Evidence for Somatic Exercises Reducing Chronic Pain:

A study published in the Journal of Bodywork and Movement Therapies in 2010 investigated the effects of a year-long somatic exercise program on chronic pain sufferers. The results showed a significant decrease in pain frequency. The intervention group, who participated in somatic exercises, experienced an 86% reduction in the number of days with pain compared to the control group [Erickson, M. A., & Shaw, L. S. (2010). The effectiveness of a mind-body movement therapy for chronic low back pain: A randomized controlled trial.

This study provides evidence that somatic exercises can be a valuable tool for managing chronic pain. It's important to note that this is a single study, but it highlights the potential benefits of this approach.

Effectiveness in Alleviating Chronic Pain

One of the primary reasons somatic exercises are effective in reducing chronic pain lies in their emphasis on flexibility, balance, and mobility. Unlike dynamic stretches commonly performed before workouts, somatic stretches involve holding stretches, which can enhance both mobility and flexibility. Additionally, practices such as tai chi and yoga, which are forms of somatic exercises, can further contribute to improving the body's flexibility and mobility.

Emotional Well-being and Mood Enhancement

Beyond physical benefits, somatic exercise can also alleviate feelings of anxiety and enhance mood by fostering a deeper understanding of the mind-body connection. Practicing somatic exercises encourage individuals to identify and address the physical manifestations of emotions, such as tension in the shoulders, headaches, or stomach discomfort, which care often associated with anxiety. By practicing somatic breathing exercises and tuning into bodily sensations, individuals can effectively manage stress responses, shifting from a state of self-preservation to one of relaxation, learning, and adaptation.

Increased Awareness of Emotions and Mind-Body Connection

Moreover, somatic exercises facilitate increased awareness and connection with one's emotions. In today's fast-paced world, many individuals may find themselves disconnected from their emotions due to constant distractions and busyness of daily life. Somatic exercises can serve as a tool to reconnect with your emotions and understand underlying emotional states that may be contributing to physical symptoms, such as chronic pain, muscle tension, joint pain, poor posture, limited range of motion, balance issues and so on.

Mindful Brain Engagement and Neuroplasticity

The mindful nature of somatic movement engages specific areas of the brain, fostering communication with various systems and organs within the body. By intentionally focusing on the subtle movements and sensations of the soma—the sensory organism encompassing beliefs, emotions, experiences, and habits—individuals can gain insights into their attitudes, behaviors, and habits. Over time, somatic exercises can effectively rewire the brain, leading to a better understanding of mindfulness, reduced pain, improved posture, and enhanced overall well-being.

Release of Chronically Tight Muscles and Improved Mobility

Incorporating mindfulness techniques into somatic movement enhances its benefits. This can help release chronically tight muscles, reduce pain, increase mobility, and improve posture. By cultivating awareness through somatic movement, individuals can develop a profound understanding of their physical and emotional states, empowering them to take control of their health and well-being.

In summary, the primary reasons for engaging in somatic exercises include their effectiveness in alleviating chronic pain, enhancing emotional well-being, fostering awareness of emotions and the mind-body connection, promoting mindful brain engagement and neuroplasticity, and improving mobility by releasing tight muscles.

Somatic exercises offer a holistic approach to health and wellness, empowering you to take control of your physical and emotional well-being. This is possible through mindful movement and self-awareness.

When Should We Do Somatic Exercise?

Engaging in somatic exercises regularly is essential for managing stress and alleviating the aftermath of trauma. Incorporating somatic exercises into your daily routine can help release accumulated stress and trauma from your body before it leads to feelings of tiredness, weakness, or chronic pain.

- **Post-Workout Cool Down**

After a workout session, somatic exercises serve as an effective cool-down method. Pandiculation, which is a form of somatic exercises that involves a stretching and yawning reflex, helps release muscle tension built up during workout sessions, improves circulation, and speeds up the recovery process. By practicing somatic exercises regularly, you can prevent tension from building up in your body, ensuring you feel ready to work out again the next day.

- **Morning and Evening Practices**

Some people prefer to start their day with somatic exercises. This helps them loosen up and feel better as they go about their daily activities. If you usually wake up feeling sore, tight, or achy, incorporating somatic exercises into your morning routine can help alleviate these symptoms and improve your overall well-being. Additionally, adding an evening practice can further enhance relaxation and promote better sleep.

- **Daily Practice for Self-Care**

Ideally, somatic exercises should be practiced every day as part of a self-care routine. Similar to brushing your teeth, daily pandiculation helps release tension built up throughout the day, preventing the gradual buildup of muscle tension. By maintaining a daily somatic practice, you can effectively manage stress, improve mobility, and enhance overall well-being.

- **Flexible Practice Duration**

The length of time for somatic practice can vary based on individual preferences and schedules. While some people set aside thirty minutes or more daily for their practice, starting with shorter durations, such as ten or fifteen minutes, can help establish a daily habit. Over time, as you experience the benefits of somatic exercises, you may find yourself practicing more frequently and for longer durations.

Avoiding Overtraining and Allowing Integration

It's important to avoid overtraining or practicing excessively in hopes of accelerating changes in the nervous system. Allowing time for new postures and movement habits to gradually integrate into the nervous system is essential for effective somatic practice. Regardless of the time spent practicing, taking the time to explore the patterns of tension in your body and relaxing during somatic exercises is key to maximizing its benefits.

By incorporating somatic exercises into your daily routine and being mindful of the timing and duration of your practice, you can effectively manage stress, alleviate chronic pain, improve mobility, and enhance overall well-being. Remember, somatic exercises should be a source of relaxation and enjoyment, helping you connect with your body and promote self-care.

How Do We Do Somatic Exercise?

Practicing somatic exercises involves a series of techniques designed to help you reconnect with your body and release stored tension. To effectively practice somatic exercises, follow these steps:

- **Selecting a Suitable Environment**

Find a calm, comfortable, and quiet space where you won't be disturbed. This could be a peaceful room in your home, an outdoor location, or anywhere you feel relaxed and at ease.

- **Incorporating Mindful Movement**

Introduce mindful movement into your practice by engaging in yoga postures, stretching, or other movements that make you feel good in your body. Pay attention to how each movement feels in your body. If emotions or feelings come up, that's okay. You don't have to judge them.

- **Resting and Reflecting After Practice**

After completing your somatic exercises, take a few moments to rest and reflect on your experience. You may notice feelings of relief, relaxation, or emotional release, which are all beneficial outcomes of the practice.

- **Consistent Practice for Effective Results**

To get the most out of somatic exercises and heal from trauma, you need to practice them regularly. Try to set aside dedicated time each day for your practice, whether it's a few minutes in the morning, during a work break, or before bedtime.

- **Personalized Experience and Listening to Your Body**

Somatic exercise is a personal practice, and everyone's experience will be different. Move at your own pace and pay attention to the signals your body gives you during the practice. If you ever feel uncomfortable or unsure, pause the exercise and return to it once you feel more comfortable.

- **Seeking Professional Guidance When Needed**

If you experience significant discomfort or emotional distress during somatic exercises, it may be beneficial to consult a qualified somatic therapist or mental health professional for personalized interventions and guidance.

By following these steps and guidelines, you can effectively practice somatic exercises to reconnect with your body, release stored tension, and promote overall well-being. Remember to move at your own pace, listen to your body, and seek professional guidance when needed to ensure a safe and beneficial practice.

How Does Somatic Exercise Affect Trauma?

A lot needs to be said here since traumatic experiences can have a profound and lasting impact on an individual's life, leading to symptoms of post-traumatic stress disorder (PTSD) or complex PTSD (CPTSD). This impact can persist for weeks, months, or even years after the event. These experiences, ranging from physical or emotional abuse to accidents or natural disasters, affect not only an individual's mental health but also their emotional well-being, physical health, and relationships.

Somatic exercises for trauma release offer an effective approach to addressing and healing from traumatic experiences. By focusing on physical movement and bodily awareness, somatic exercises help individuals process and release traumatic emotions stored in their bodies, allowing them to regain a sense of control over their bodies and minds. Regular practice of somatic exercises can promote healing and resilience in the face of trauma, providing a powerful tool for recovery from emotional wounds.

In addition to addressing trauma, somatic exercises offer numerous benefits for overall health and well-being. By intentionally listening to the body and becoming more aware of physical sensations, individuals can regulate their emotions and reduce the impact of everyday stress, fostering a deeper connection with their bodies and promoting self-care.

After experiencing trauma:

Trauma can make you feel disconnected from your body and mind, which can affect how you feel overall. And that's where somatic exercises come in.

These exercises aim at bridging this gap, allowing you to regain a sense of wholeness and start your healing journey. By focusing on sensations, breathing, and movements, somatic exercises help you become more conscious of your body and the present moment, encouraging you to listen to your body and honor your needs.

Integrating somatic exercises with traditional therapy and support systems can create a holistic recovery plan that promotes emotional management and equips you to navigate triggers and setbacks with greater ease and resilience. By acknowledging and understanding the impact of trauma on both the mind and body, you can begin your healing journey, connect with your body, release stored emotional and physical tension, and restore balance through somatic exercises. Though the journey towards healing may not always be easy, being patient and compassionate with yourself can help you gradually heal from the inside out. Somatic exercises for trauma release can provide a safe space for healing and growth.

Nutrition and trauma recovery

Imagine some sort of worrying and cramping feeling in your stomach right before a big exam or presentation. Or imagine feeling sick, anxious, and restless after eating a lot of junk the previous night. These are just some examples of how your gut might be connected to your entire body.

This may sound unbelievable, but there are many examples to back this up. You've probably experienced some of them. Think of it this way: there are countless microorganisms in our gut with different functions. Some break down your food and aid digestion, some help absorb the digested food, and some produce neurotransmitters that influence mood, sleep, emotions, and stress response.

These microorganisms are like us—they need food for energy, they need rest after working, and they don't like anything that puts pressure on them. They also don't like certain foods because they are hard to break down. That's why you feel hungover after a wild night. Unhealthy foods, irregular eating, and sleeping patterns can throw them off balance, bringing about a reaction. A great illustration is earthworms; they like to burrow into the soil, but when you add a bit of salt to their path, they move irrationally because salt is harmful to their cells.

Stressful events and our reactions to such events (which could include stress eating, drinking, or eating at odd hours) impact the flora of our guts, sending mixed signals that can alter our moods and sleep.

How Diet Affects Mood and Anxiety

You need to know that what you eat can affect your mental health. It's important to understand how this happens and how you can make better food choices as this helps to improve your mood and reduce anxiety. Here's how your food can influence your mood and anxiety levels:

1. **Neurotransmitter Production:** the microorganisms or microbiome in your gut has a vital task of producing neurotransmitters in your body. Neurotransmitters act just like the blood moving through the body and sending absorbed food and fluid to cells where they are

needed. Neurotransmitters don't use blood, but they send messages from nerve cells to target cells chemically, and that is why they are called the chemical messengers of the body. Some examples of neurotransmitters are;

    a. **Serotonin:** its role includes mood regulation.

    b. **GABA:** this neurotransmitter is associated with mood regulation and stress relief.

2. **Inflammation and Stress Response:** Scientists have associated inflammation in the body with various health issues. Some health issues that could arise as a result of chronic inflammation are anxiety, depression, and even heart disease. But how does inflammation happen? How does it cause health challenges?

Inflammations are the body's response to traumatic events such as cuts or wounds. At one point or another, you might have had an injury from a kitchen accident or a bad fall that gave you bruises all over.? Do you remember how these wounds heal after a while? That healing was made possible by inflammation.

They are like a repair crew that are only awaken when there's an injury. When white blood cells notice any injury, they run to the rescue, induce inflammation, and start the healing process. However, there are some cases when inflammation do not come as a result of an injury but they come when you eat some kinds of food.

You don't want inflammation awaken when there's no injury; they cause an imbalance that can affect your health. Sugary foods and processed food can trigger inflammation, but foods like fruits and vegetables can help reduce inflammation.

3. **Blood Sugar Regulation:** You should know by now that what you eat can affect your blood sugar. Diabetes tops the list and it can lead to several health challenges. One such health challenge is stroke. Excess sugar in your blood can also lead to anxiety and impact your mood. Refined carbohydrates and sugary food and drinks can spike and crash the sugar levels in your blood and this can cause an irritable feeling, increased anxiety, and fatigue. A diet you can try out if you want to keep a balanced blood sugar level is a food rich in lean protein, healthy fats, and complex carbohydrates. An example of such is quinoa salad with avocado and grilled chicken. Such foods help maintain stable blood sugar levels and promote emotional stability.

4. **Foods are memory triggers:** Your tongue is one of your sense organs and the deal with sense organs is that they are memory banks. You can smell a strange perfume on the bus, and you are taken back twenty years from when you first experienced it. Taste is like this as well, you taste a food, and memories about this taste and food bring back memories. Memories can also determine our moods, so foods can trigger a difficult situation that spikes your anxiety or triggers a traumatic experience.

Nourishing Foods for Regulating Your Nervous System

Now that you know how your food affects your gut and brain, let's look at some healthy foods that can help keep your nervous system strong and manage anxiety. These foods act like a nutritious therapy, helping you take care of your body and mental health.

You want to include the following;

- **Prebiotics and Probiotics:** Prebiotics are food for the microbiomes in your gut, while probiotics are the actual bacteria that contribute to the health of the gut. Fruits, vegetables, and whole grains are rich in prebiotics and are very good for your gut health. And remember these food substances are also great for a balanced blood sugar.
- **Omega-3 Fatty Acids:** These are abundant in flaxseeds, walnuts, and in some fatty fish. They are great for reducing inflammation and improving your mood.
- **B vitamins:** These vitamins are important for the production of neurotransmitters in the body. You can get healthy amounts of this vitamin in lentils, whole grains, and some leafy greens.
- **Magnesium:** Magnesium is a mineral that promotes sleep, relaxation, and calmness. Nuts, seeds, avocados, and leafy greens are rich in magnesium and can help you get that calming effect when you eat.

Tips for Creating a Healthy Diet that Can Be Therapeutic for You and Your Body.

1. Prioritize whole grains, fresh fruits, and vegetables. You might want to consider lean proteins and other whole food sources.
2. Include healthy fats from foods like avocados, nuts, and olive oil. They support hormone regulation and brain function.

3. Drink enough water. Water keeps everything ticking, so make sure you are taking enough water whether it's during meals or in between meals.
4. Avoid eating out as much as you can, especially junk. When you cook at home, you have many options to choose from and you can always avoid processed food.
5. Pay attention to your meal portions. Don't overeat, pay attention to the cues your body is giving you about hunger and fullness.

Take care of your gut and you've taken a great leap toward improving your physical and mental health.

Trauma recovery exercises

Before you start, engage in this 5-Minute Meditation

Grounding Before Healing:

Introduction (1 minute):

- Take a moment to find a cozy seated position on a chair or the floor. Close your eyes or soften your gaze.

- Take a few deep breaths through your nose, filling your belly with air. Slowly breathe out through your mouth, letting go of any tension.

- Notice how your body feels right now. Are there any areas that feel tight or uncomfortable? Simply observe without judgment.

Body Scan (2 minutes):

- Starting with your feet, slowly bring your attention to each body part. Notice the sensations in your toes, the soles of your feet, and your ankles.

- Move up your legs through your knees, thighs, and hips. Feel the contact between your body and the chair or floor.

- Bring your awareness to your lower back, abdomen, chest, and upper back. Notice your heartbeat, your breath rising and falling.

- Focus on your shoulders, arms, hands, and fingers. Gently wiggle your fingers and notice any tingling or warmth.

- Bring your attention to your neck, throat, and face. Relax your jaw, soften your eyes, and smooth your forehead.

Grounding (1 minute):

- Imagine a gentle magnetic force drawing your feet toward the center of the earth. Feel yourself being pulled down, grounding you and creating a sense of calm. Feel them anchoring you, providing stability and support.

- Visualize warm, comforting energy flowing through those roots, filling your body with strength and calm.

- Take a few more deep breaths, feeling the connection to the earth below you.

Closing (1 minute):

- Gently bring your awareness back to the room around you. Pay attention to the sounds you can hear and the smells you can detect.

- When you're ready, slowly open your eyes, taking a moment to adjust to your surroundings.

- Carry this sense of stability with you as you move into your somatic exercises.

Additional Notes:

- Use this meditation regularly, not just before the exercises.

- If any of the exercises you have planned for the day involve some level of movement, you can add a gentle stretch at the end of your meditation to prepare your body.

Now, let's get into the exercises...

40+ somatic Exercises with Detailed and Basic Instructions

Grounding

Grounding exercises help center and anchor you to the present moment, diverting your mind from past events that cause pain and distress. These exercises are particularly beneficial if you are experiencing anxiety, flashbacks, or symptoms of dissociation. Here are some grounding techniques you can try:

- **Run Water Over Your Hands**: Place your hands under running cold water. Focus on the sensation of the temperature on each part of your hand, from your wrist to your nails. Switch to warm water and notice how the sensation changes. Repeat this for a few minutes until you feel calmer.

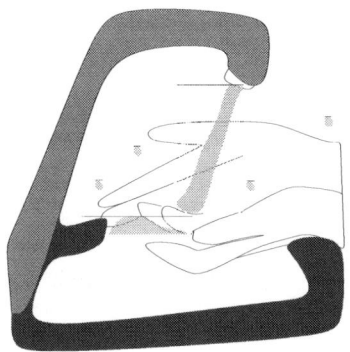

- **Focus on Your Breathing**: Control your inhalation and exhalation by inhaling to the count of four and exhaling to the count of four. You can also repeat a positive word after each inhalation, such as "safe," "easy," or "love."

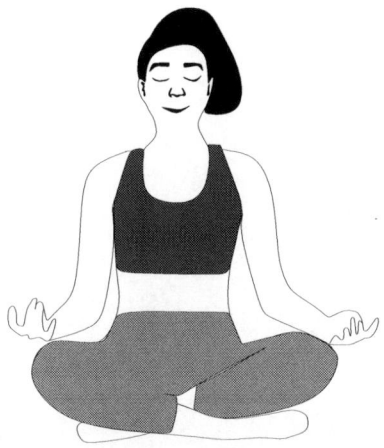

- **Play a 'Categories' Game**: Choose a letter and think of different categories of things, like cities, states, or dogs, that begin with that letter. Identify at least five objects for each category before switching to a new letter.
- **Move Your Body**: Engage in movements that feel comfortable to you, such as jumping, stretching, dancing, or jogging in place. Pay

attention to how each part of your body feels by conducting a body scan from your toes to your face.

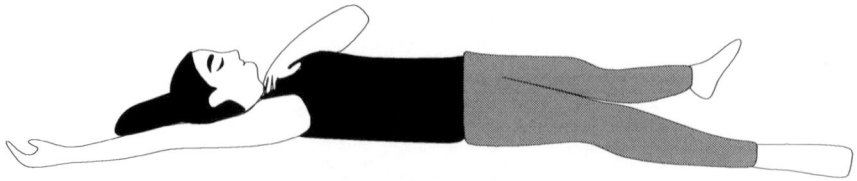

- **Tense and Relax Your Body**: Press your feet to the ground as hard as you can for a few seconds, then release and notice the sensation in your feet. Alternatively, squeeze the arms of your chair tightly and then relax slowly.

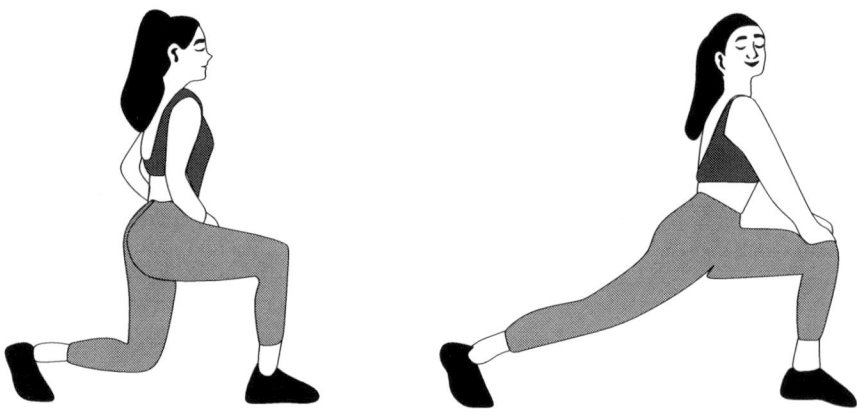

Self-regulation

Emotional self-regulation involves guiding yourself through your emotions to shift gears when they lead to distress. In somatic therapy, self-regulation focuses on the nervous system.

Unresolved trauma can result in dysregulation of the autonomic nervous system, leading to a heightened state of alertness. This can cause you to react to everyday stress and events in ways connected to your past trauma. The following are activities you can carry out in self-regulation:

- **Hug Yourself**: Cross your right arm over your chest, placing your hand near your heart, and then cross your left arm, placing your left hand on your right shoulder. According to Levine, this can make you feel contained and safe. Hold the hug for as long as you need.

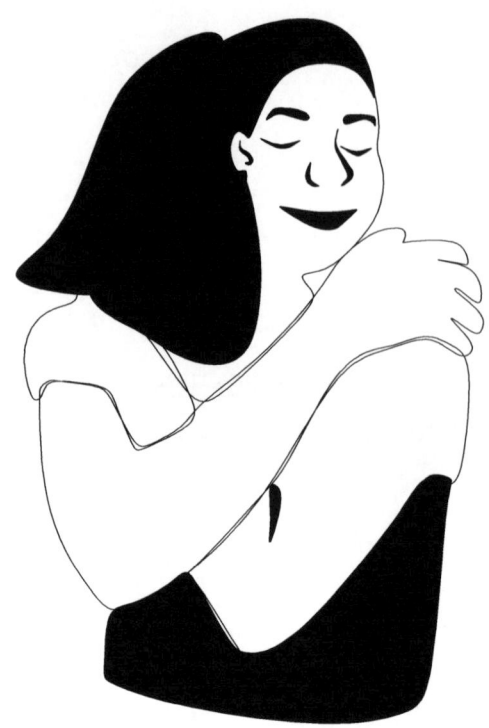

- **Tap or Squeeze Your Body**: Tap your body from your feet to your head using your hand in a cupping position. Alternatively, try squeezing different parts of your body. This will help your body recognize its boundaries, giving you a sense of containment and safety.

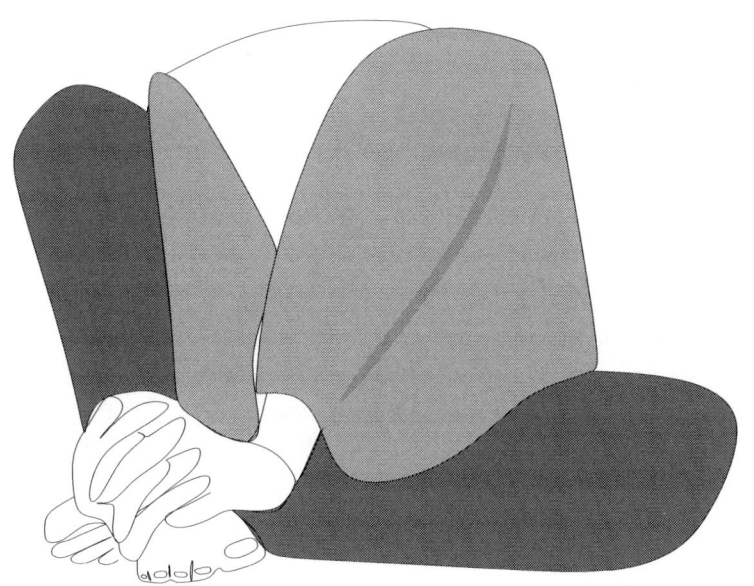

Resourcing and Visualization

Resourcing means focusing on certain body sensations that can help change how you feel. Although this can be a bit complicated and may be easier with a therapist's help, there are exercises you can try at home to get started. These exercises can support any professional treatment you're receiving.

- **Create a Safe Place in Your Mind**: Recall a time and place where you felt safe and happy. Alternatively, envision a new safe place, focusing on its colors, smells, and textures. Immerse yourself in this mental space, feeling the comfort it provides.
- **Think About Your Loved Ones**: Reflect on people who bring you peace and comfort. Look at their pictures or recall shared memories to evoke positive emotions.

Body Scans

Described by Candela Brower as "active meditation," body scans can help you relax.

- **Get Comfortable**: Sit or lie down in a relaxed position and close your eyes.
- **Focus on Your Lower Body**: Pay attention to the sensations in your feet, ankles, knees, thighs, and pelvis. Identify temperature, pressure, tension, and other sensations. When you notice tension, take a deep breath and exhale to release it. Move on to the next body part once you feel relaxed.

- **Move to Your Upper Body**: Continue the process, including internal organs like the stomach, lungs, and heart.
- **Focus on Your Neck, Head, and Face**: Conclude by paying attention to these areas, noting any sensation.

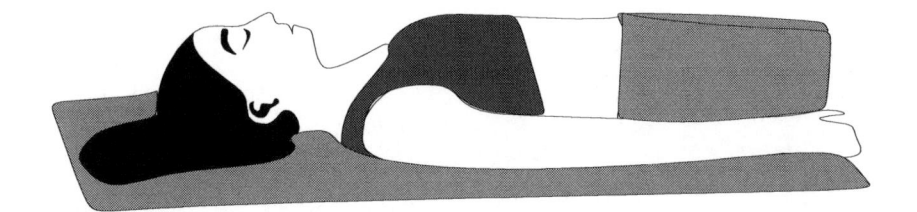

Diaphragmatic Breathing

This exercise activates your body's relaxation response by promoting deep breathing into the diaphragm rather than shallow chest breathing.

- **Find a Comfortable Position**: Sit or lie down comfortably.
- **Place Your Hands**: Place one hand on your belly and the other on your chest.
- **Breathe In**: Inhale slowly through your nose, allowing your belly to rise while keeping the hand on your chest as still as possible.
- **Breathe Out**: Exhale slowly through your mouth or nose, allowing your belly to fall.
- **Repeat**: Continue this deep breathing exercise several times.

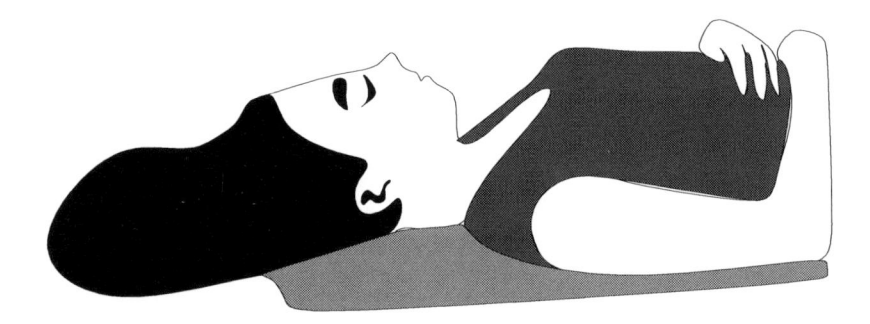

Somatic Yoga

Somatic yoga involves practicing traditional yoga poses with heightened attention to internal body sensations. It's recommended to practice this with a certified somatic yoga instructor.

In this exercise, practitioners are encouraged to explore movements slowly and with intention, paying absolute attention or focus to how each of the movement feels rather than striving for a certain end posture. This approach gives room for individuals to reduce tension, improve flexibility and enhance bodily awareness which has the ability to develop a greater understanding of your physical and emotional experiences.

- **Choose a Yoga Pose**: Select a yoga pose you feel comfortable with.
- **Focus on Body Sensations**: Move into the pose mindfully, paying close attention to how each movement feels.
- **Hold the Pose:** Maintain the pose for a few breaths while remaining aware of your bodily sensations.

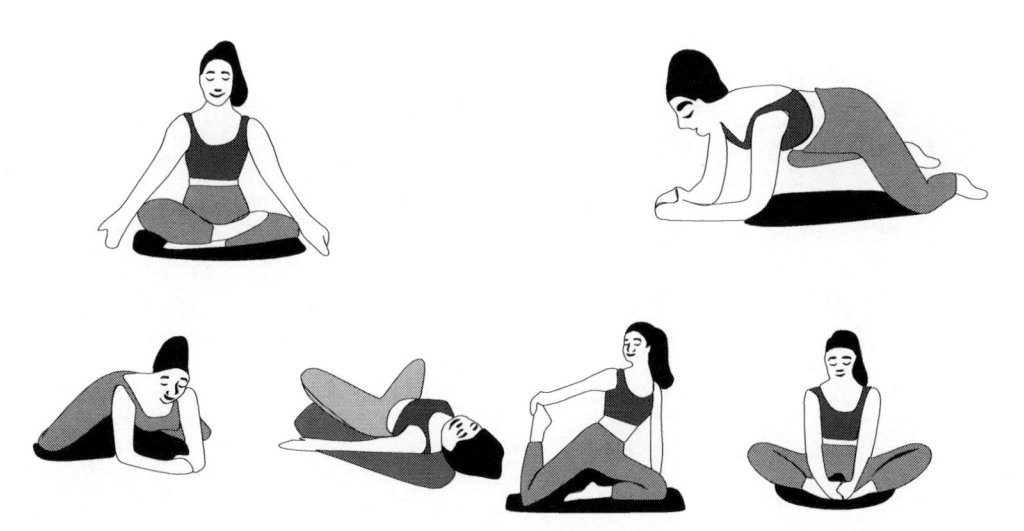

Progressive Muscle Relaxation (PMR)

PMR involves systematically tensing and then relaxing different muscle groups to induce relaxation. Practice this technique mindfully.

- **Start with Your Toes**: Begin at one end of your body, like your toes.
- **Tense the Muscles**: Tighten the muscles in that area as much as you can for about five seconds.
- **Relax the Muscles**: Release the tension and notice the sensation of relaxation.
- **Move On:** Proceed to the next muscle group, such as your legs, and repeat the process.

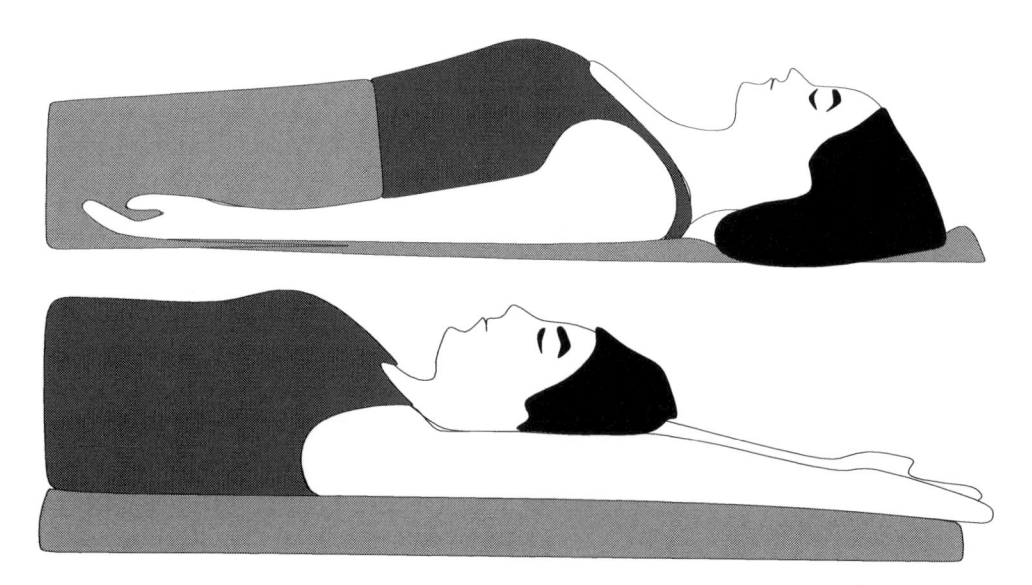

The Voo Breath

The Voo Breath is a vocal exercise designed to stimulate your vagus nerve, promoting a sense of calm and relaxation.

- **Find a Comfortable Position**: Sit in a chair or on the floor in a comfortable position.
- **Focus on the Present**: Pay attention to your bodily sensations and your breath as you inhale and exhale.
- **Take a Deep Breath In**: Inhale deeply.
- **Exhale with a 'Voo' Sound**: As you exhale, make a 'voo' sound and sustain the vowel for as long as possible, feeling the vibration in your abdomen and chest.
- **Repeat**: Practice this several times.

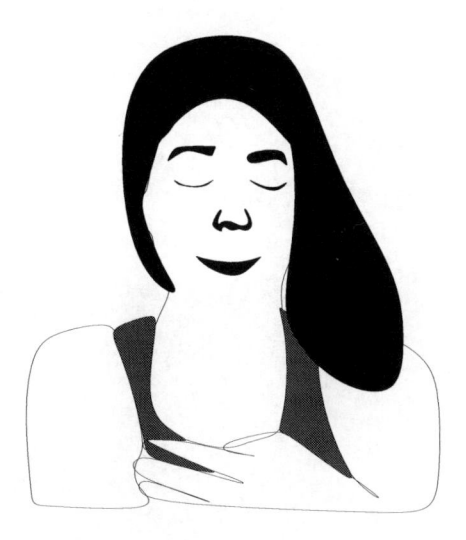

Shake Out the Tension

This somatic exercise helps release physical tension and excess energy caused by stress.

- **Find a Comfortable Place**: Choose a comfortable place to stand.
- **Start Shaking**: Begin shaking your body starting with your hands, gradually incorporating your arms, torso, and legs. Imagine shaking off dust or sand from your body.
- **Shake and Wind Down**: Continue shaking for a few minutes, then gradually slow down to bring your body back to balance.
- **Notice the Difference**: Pay attention to how your body feels after shaking.

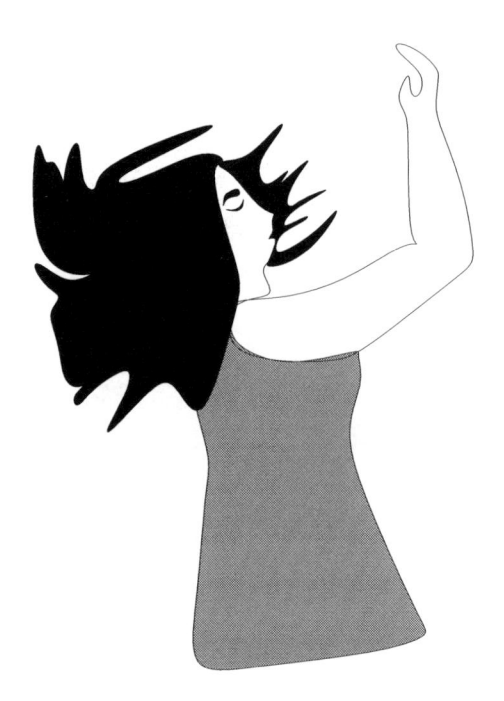

Walking Meditation

This combines physical movement with mindfulness practice.

- **Walk Slowly**: Start walking at a slow, comfortable pace.
- **Focus on Your Senses**: Focus on how your feet feel on the ground, how your arms and legs move, and the rhythm of your breath.
- **Stay Present**: If your thoughts drift to something else (maybe something pops up in your mind), gently refocus on the feeling of walking and what's happening right now.

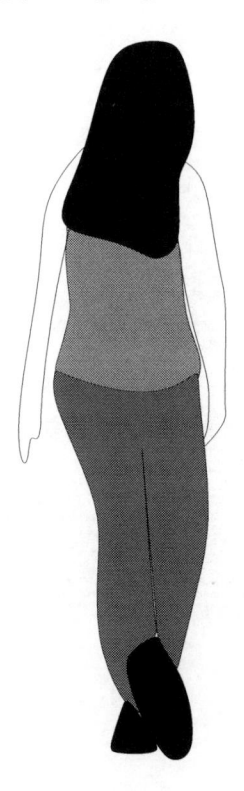

Sensory Awareness

This exercise promotes heightened awareness of your sensory experiences.

- **Find a Quiet Place**: Sit or lie down in a quiet place.
- **Close Your Eyes and Breathe**: Take a few deep breaths with your eyes closed.
- **Tune into Your Senses**: Focus on what you can hear, smell, feel, taste, and see (with your eyes closed).

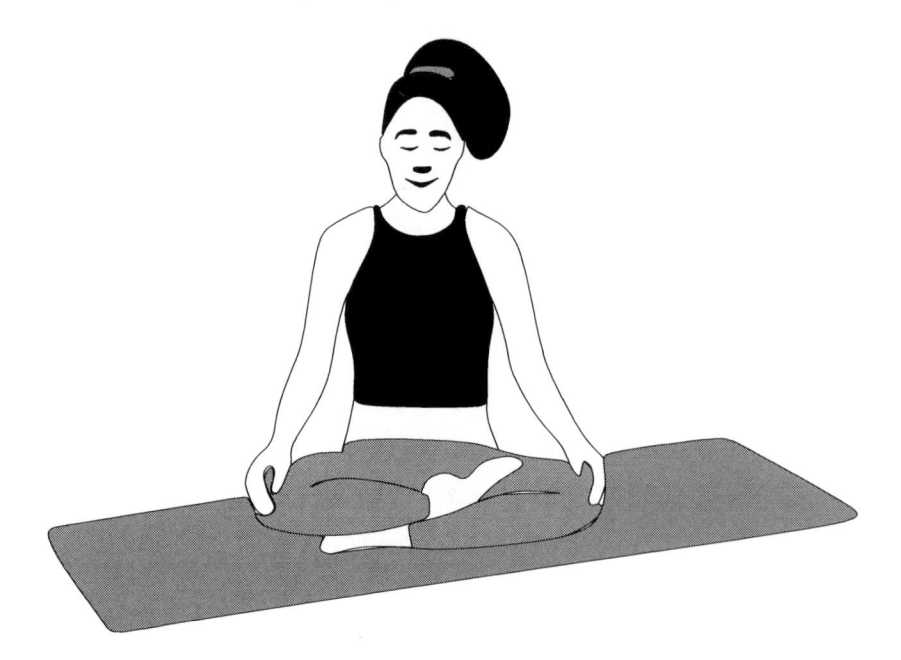

Felt Sense

This exercise enhances your ability to tune in to and articulate your felt sense which is also known as the sensations you have throughout your entire body, both subtly and prominently. If it follows a painful or traumatic experience, it can be difficult at times to retain the connection you have with your body at a time.

There is often the need to actively relearn how to have those feelings of bodily sensations in order to feel safe occupying your body. At first, you may find it strange, abnormal and challenging to do the reconnection, but Felt Sense is a common exercise which will help you reconnect with your body.

During the exercises, if you find yourself connecting back to the part of your body that is connected or linked to trauma and it becomes uncomfortable, it is very good and advisable to do any of these two: It is either you gently redirect your awareness towards a neutral or relaxed part of the body, or give thoughtful resources to that place. For instance, you say "I am here for you", "I am with you", "I love you", and so on, in effect using your awareness to extend an empathic connection with that part of your body.

- **Get Comfortable**: Sit or lie down comfortably.
- **Describe Sensations**: Start from your toes and work your way up, describing the sensations in each part of your body. Pay attention to the part that brings the most sensation and use descriptive words like cold, tense, warm, gentle, aching, stabbing, etc.
- **Ask Either/Or Questions**: Pose questions like "Is it more tense or relaxed?" or "Does it feel heavy or light?"

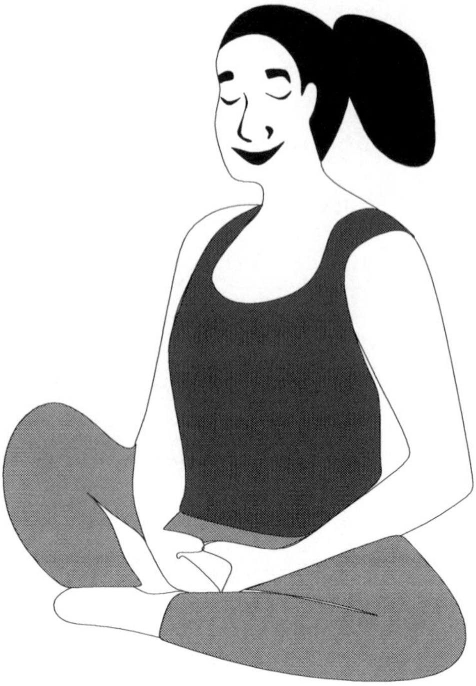

Heel Drops

This exercise helps mobilize your body's adrenaline and cortisol, releasing and discharging this energy.

- **Stand and Focus**: Stand without focusing on anything in particular.
- **Raise to Toes and Drop to Heels**: Slowly raise up to your toes and then drop back down to your heels, imagining a weight dropping through your heels with each drop. Let it make a loud thud and give yourself the chance or permission to make noise and take up space.
- **Repeat**: Continue this movement rhythmically, allowing stress and tension to release from your body.

Bring your focus and attention to the aftermath of this movement and the effects it has had on your hips and lower back; maybe it feels as though the jolt loosens them. Try to make them relax, and every time you return to a standing position, imagine that the stress and tension are making their way out of your body.

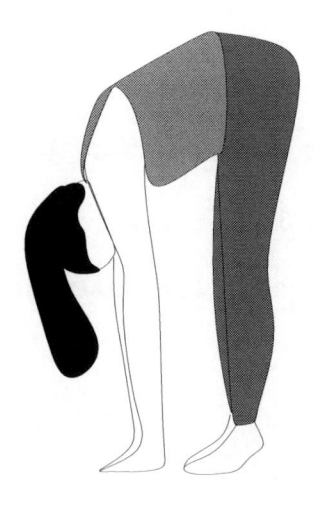

Recalling a Kindness

This exercise encourages you to focus on positive memories when you were on the receiving end of an act of kindness. The memories can help you in nurturing positive emotions and feelings and recognitions within your body as a way to remove and do away with the negative ones. Doing so will help you develop the ability to soothe yourself and bring your nervous system to a state of calmness by gaining from your positive emotions associated with memories.

- **Recall a Kind Moment**: Remember a time when someone was kind to you. Focus on the details of the moment, such as tone, touch, voice, and action. Try to remember what the person used to soothe or comfort you.
- **Notice Sensations**: Pay attention to the sensations in your body as you recall this memory.
- **Recall Emotions**: Remember the emotions you felt then and notice how you feel now as you recall them.

If a negative aspect of the event comes to mind, set that part in an imaginary safe and come back to the sensory aspects of this memory of kindness.

As you conclude, notice the sensations in your body and your total experience now, in comparison to when you started the exercise.

Body Mapping

This exercise helps you visually observe, describe, and draw what you notice or feel is happening in your body. It is a body awareness and mindfulness tool.

- **Prepare Materials**: Get a sheet of paper, a marker, pen, or colored pencils.
- **Draw Your Body Outline**: Sketch an outline representing your body. You really don't have to be an artist or be able to draw perfectly. Just sketch out something that represents your body.
- **Tune Inward**: Take a deep breath and exhale fully. Close your eyes and place a hand on your heart or wherever feels comfortable for you.
- **Notice Your Body**: Ask yourself what you notice in your body that needs attention. Are there any images, feelings, physical sensations or point of construction?

Draw: Draw intuitivelyy the areas that are giving response. Don't overthink this part, just allow yourself flow with it. Make a sketch of the areas where you notice something is present. You can make use of colors, shapes, or symbols and let yourself express what you notice.

Observe: Once complete, take a moment to observe what is present. You may even take note of where you want to give more attention. Just observe what is there.

Title: When you are done, give your body a title that best represents this body-focused experience.

Draw in here

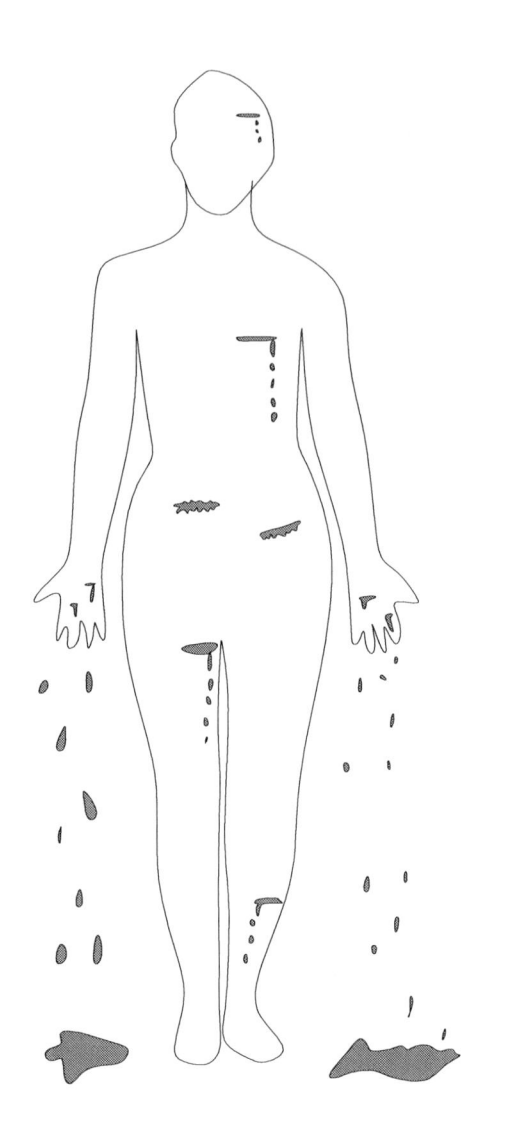

Self-Holding

This exercise helps in calming the nervous system and it does this by promoting reintegration with your body. It enhances body awareness and provides a comforting environment for the nervous system to recognize stability. The objective is to visualize the body as a container, establishing a sense of personal boundaries. Try to take note of all the feelings as they pass through you as if you are watching a flowing stream, noting colors, energy, shapes, motion, and sounds.

- Choose to close or keep your eyes open based on your comfort.
- Sit or lie down.
- Place one open palm on your forehead and the other hand on your heart.
- Focus on the sensation of the hand on your forehead. Note its texture, temperature, and any other sensations.
- Similarly, focus on the hand on your heart.
- Reflect on your observations.

Did you feel safe in your body during this exercise?

Were there moments you didn't feel traumatized?

Can you envision feeling safe in your body in the future?

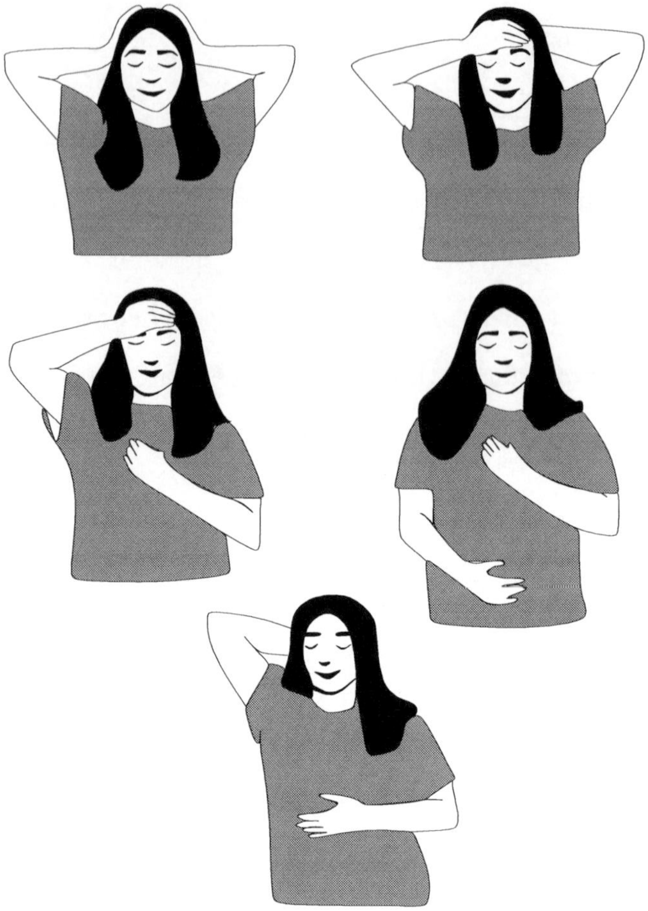

Orienting

This exercise involves grounding yourself by actively sensing your environment. By doing so, you signal to your nervous system that you are safe and present in the current moment. This increases awareness of your existence in your surroundings and promotes a sense of security.

Look around and find something you like to look at. Make sure it makes you feel good or at least doesn't bother you.

As you orient yourself to the moment, focus on what happens in your body. If you do not find anything around you that you are naturally drawn to, you can give yourself some detail to look for. This can be you searching for a particular color, pattern or shape you can orient to touch and sound well.

Closed Loop Connection to Your Body

This technique fosters a feeling of containment, support, connection, and presence within your body, especially during moments of distress. It helps calm the nervous system by reinforcing the idea that your body is yours alone, and no one else's.

- Cross your arms and tuck your hands under the opposite armpits.
- Cross your ankles and, if comfortable, squeeze them slightly.
- Lower your head towards your body slowly.
- Breathe slowly and deeply for 30 to 60 seconds, or until you feel calm, comfortable and supported.

Wave Breathing

This exercise promotes relaxation and stabilizes breathing by using imagery and visualization. It can be done while standing or sitting.

- Begin by noticing your breathing. Relax your body and gently sway back and forth with your eyes closed.
- Focus on the movement in your spine and feel the weight shift throughout your body.
- Visualize a gentle wave expanding as you inhale and cresting and falling as you exhale.
- With each breath, visualize the wave growing larger in your mind.
- Inhale deeply through your nose, imagining the wave expanding.
- Exhale and visualize the wave crashing onto the beach.
- Continue breathing in this rhythmic pattern, visualizing waves of varying sizes, until you feel a sense of calmness and stillness throughout your body.

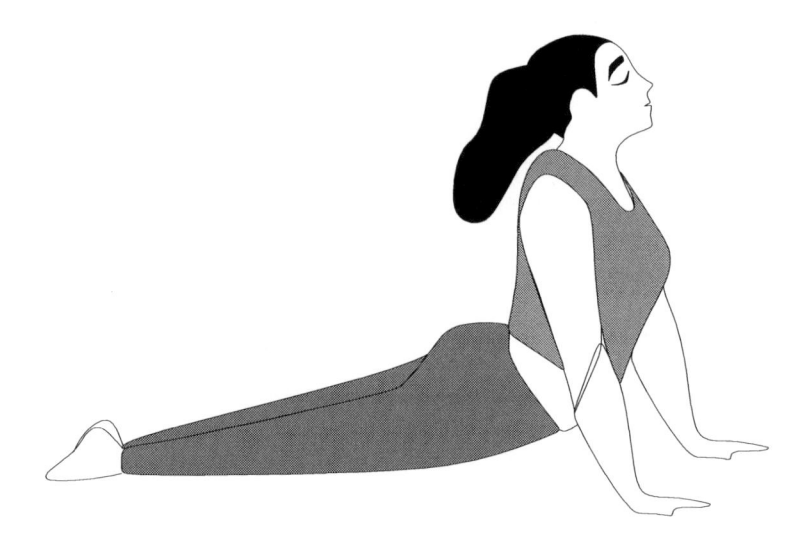

Pendulation

This somatic exercise involves alternating between states of tension and relaxation. It helps the body identify and appreciate contrasts between different physical and emotional states, fostering a deeper understanding and acceptance of feelings and emotions.

- Consciously tighten and release each muscle group, noting shifting sensations.
- Track your mood on a scale of 1 to 10 throughout the day, observing its fluctuations.
- Take five deep belly breaths when caught ruminating to center yourself.
- Go for an outdoor walk, paying attention to changing thoughts and feelings.

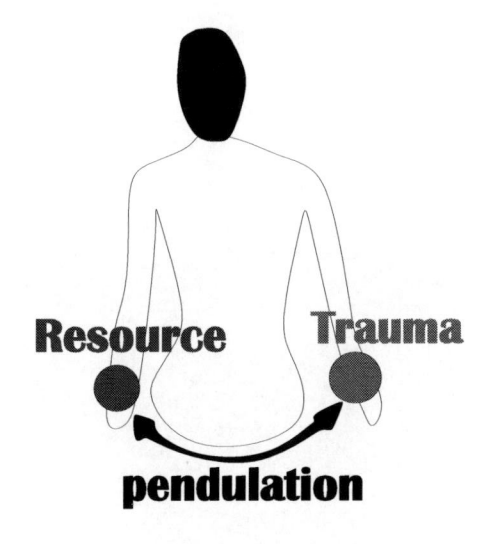

Containment With Safe Touch

This nurturing technique uses compassionate physical touch to establish a sense of stability and safety, helping contain overwhelming emotions and fostering internal support and self-compassion.

- Wrap your arms around yourself in a tender hug and apply gentle pressure. Feel your breath rise and fall against the embrace.
- Cup your hands together, cradling them together. Bring them up to the centre of you heart and feel their soothing warmth as you take deep breaths.
- Rest on a pillow or stuffed animal where the tension is held in your body. You can be relieved through its softness.
- Lay a soft weighted blanket over your torso or lap. Its calming pressure can work its magic, containing difficult emotions.

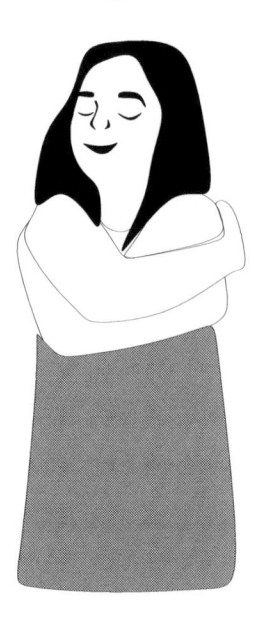

Rhythmic Movement

This exercise centers the body and mind by encouraging you to move in tune with your body's innate rhythms freely. It is not like pendulation which oscillates between tension and relaxation. This instinctive motion aligns you with the natural rhythms you carry within.

- Let your body sway gently from side to side or front to back, falling into an instinctive, flowing dance.
- Rock your torso, head nodding forward and backward, releasing the tension stored up in the spine.
- Walk at an easy pace, coordinating arm swings with each step to find your natural rhythm.

The thing is, do not force any motion. Instead, tune into rhythms that feel good in your body. Move in ways that are intuitive, easy and calming.

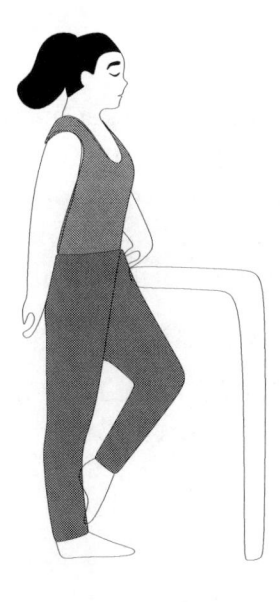

Body Movement Technique

Gentle movements harmonize the body and mind. It releases all the stored up tension in your body and makes you feel more at home in your skin

Practice therapeutic yoga postures thoughtfully. Don't move forcefully but thoughtfully.

To express emotions in a way that is free of judgement, dance freely. Use your body as a guide.

Targeted stretches for tight areas. Tension melts away with breath and gentle movement.

Shoulder and neck rolls relieve you of the tension hunching over screens and desks.

Shake out your body for about thirty minutes to clear the tension that are stuck. It really works.

Jumping jacks or jogging on the spot to get energy moving again.

Walking meditations are where you consciously take note of each step and sensation. Being in nature brings about peace.

Ensure you start slowly and pay close attention to how movements feel, not perfect form. You will feel more balanced and integrated over time.

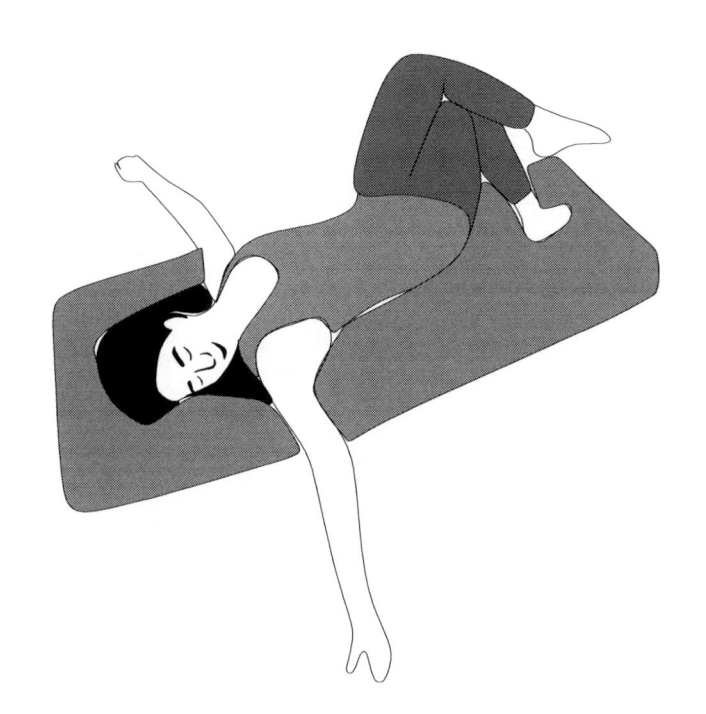

Bioenergy

This refers to the vibration, warmth, and current animating your body systems, which can be constrained by chronic stress, poor posture, and repressed emotions.

Perform expansive stretches to remove congestion from the torso and increase energy flow.

Try full-body shakes to break up every stagnant energy and dissipate chronic tension.

Learn qigong or tai chi to optimize bioenergy circulation.

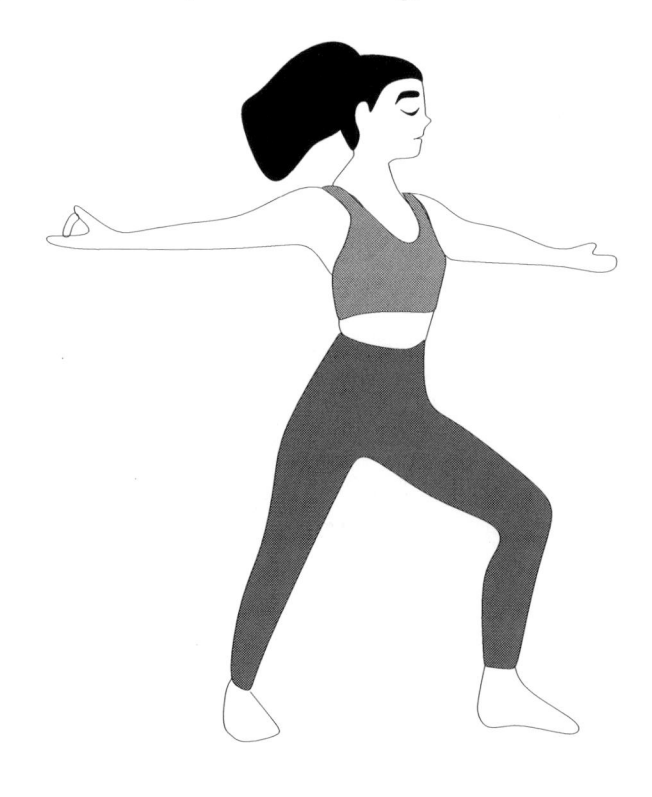

Butterfly Hug

This is a comforting somatic exercise to practice when feeling down or sad. If you are feeling down or going through sadness, and you seek comfort and soothing, butterfly hug is one of the best somatic exercises that you can practice.

You can start by interlacing your thumbs, bringing your hands across your chest and allowing your fingers reach towards your shoulders.

Know that there is no right or wrong way to do this.

Allow yourself to settle in feeling the comforting and soothing sensation in your arms.

When you are ready, gently alternatively tap your hands in a rhythmic motion that you are comfortable with.

Do this for as long as you desire. It is very important to know that this practice can result into a significant emotional release. If you find yourself becoming emotionally or at the verge of tears, it is okay.

Just allow yourself to embrace those feelings.

On the other hand, if the technique simply gives you the sensation of soothing without bringing up strong emotions, continue for as long as you find it good and beneficial.

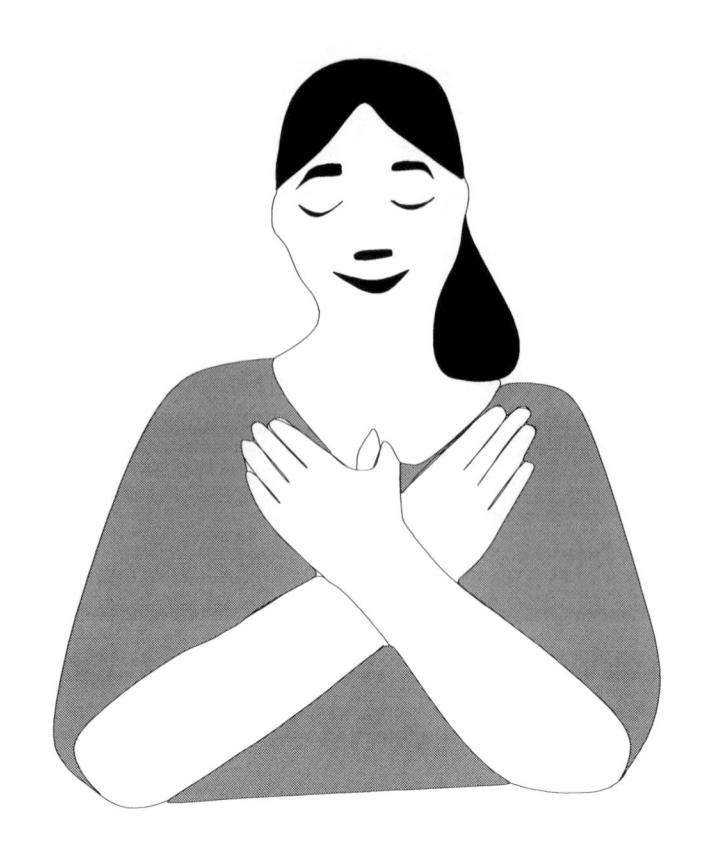

Goddess Pose

This exercise is a grounding pose suitable for everyone, regardless of gender. If you don't want to call it that as a male, you can give it another name.

Turn your feet out and bring your hands, let's say to heart center if you are into yoga.

Inhale as you come down, allowing your knees go out.

Exhale, letting your arms go up to the ceiling.

There's no definite pace, so do this at the pace you are comfortable with and that you feel is good for you.

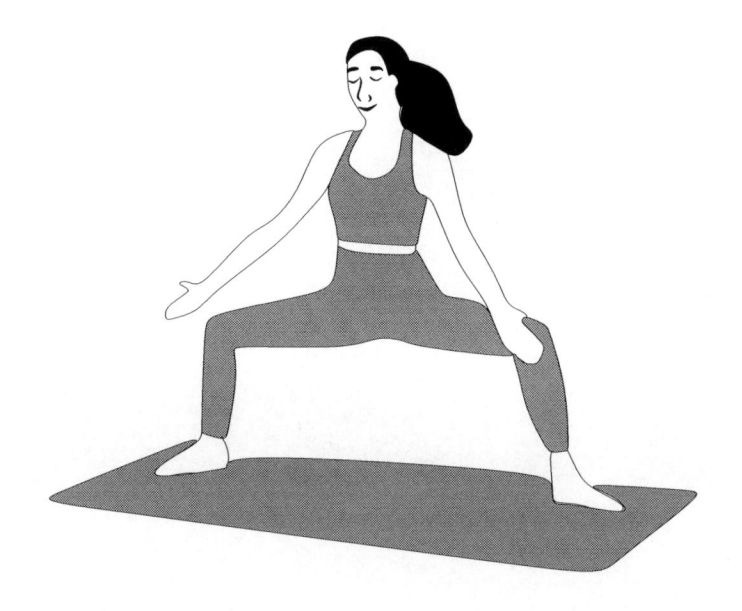

Wipe Away

This is a technique to release frustration.

Find a good and comfortable position that suits your body.

Imagine wiping away frustrations.

Bend over and make sure the posture is a comfortable one.

As you wipe away, allow those feelings you are experiencing flow through your body.

You can give an increase to the intensity of this movement as you become more and more at ease.

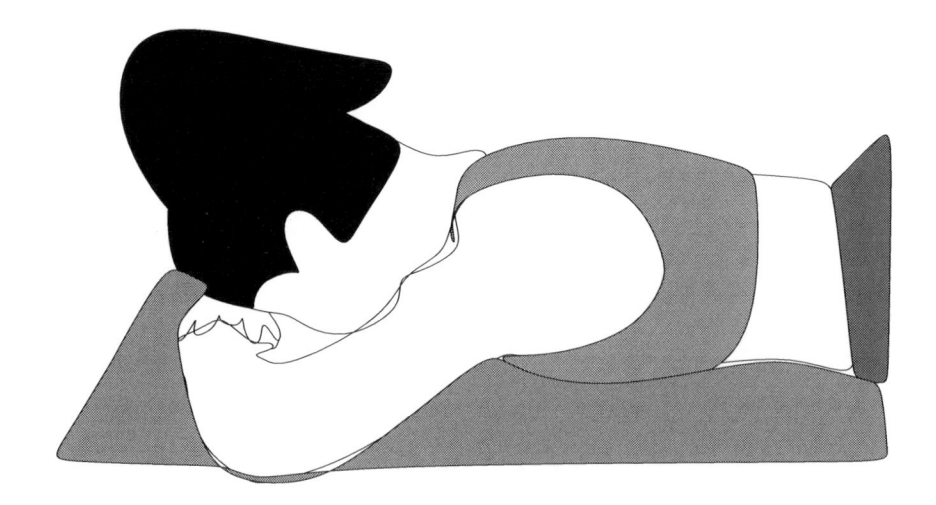

Shaking

This is a somatic technique to release pent-up energy. It is an idea reminiscent of the way wild animals deal with fight-or-flight responses. They would shake (literally) off the stress and swiftly return to a state of homeostasis.

So if you are feeling frustrated, and want to release some pent-up energy, do the following:

Shake your body vigorously. Shake your body as much as you need

Take a moment to settle.

Then, take time to connect with yourself and observe the sensations in your body.

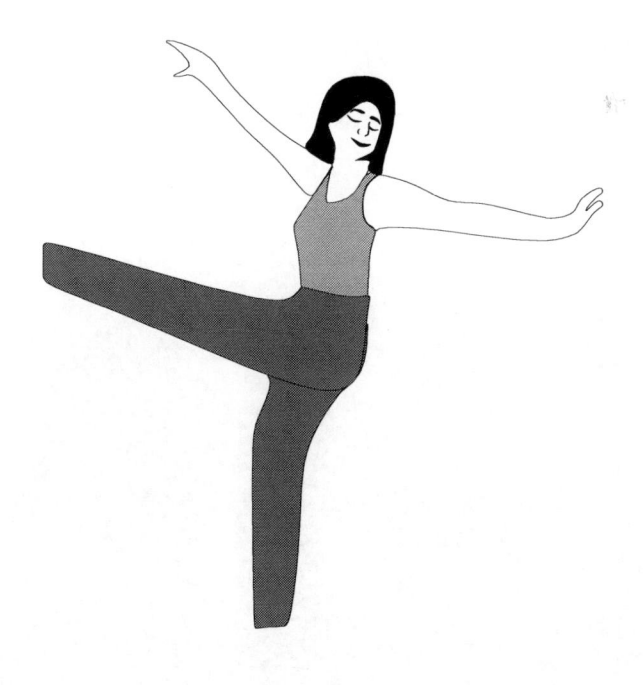

When You Felt Most Like Yourself

This exercise will keep you grounded, promoting emotional and nervous system regulation.

Notice your overall experience for a moment.

Recall a time in the last twenty-four hours when you felt like yourself or the person you would hope to be more of the time. You can extend the time frame if nothing comes to mind from the last day.

As you remember this event in a detailed way, like it was happening again, take note of what happens in your body presently and your five senses, too. Notice what happens with them.

Try to recall another time you most felt like yourself or the person you would like or aspire to be, this time within the last several weeks.

Again, as you remember the details almost as if it was happening again, notice what happens in your body presently.

What do you notice now about your overall experience?

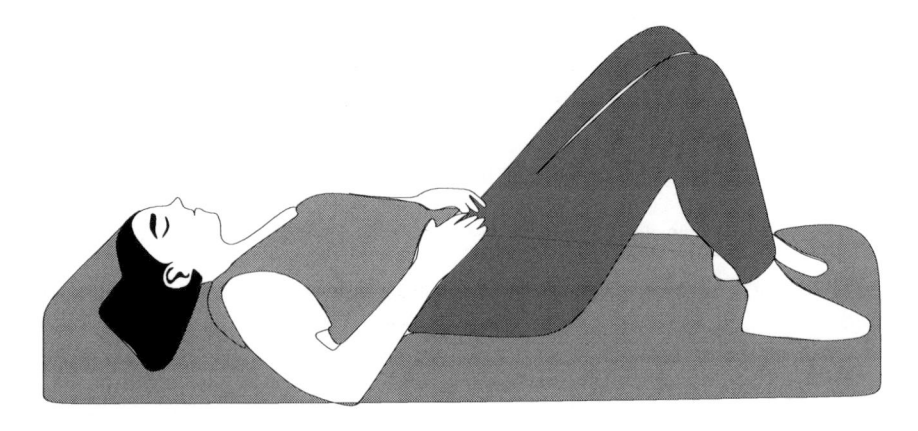

Notice Your Current Physical Comfort

A technique to focus on physical comfort. Tune out your circumstances for just a moment and bring your attention to your physical comfort in this technique. Take your time with each of these steps in a way that you spend at least one minute with the entire exercise.

Sit in a chair and take a moment, noticing your overall experience.

Move your feet on the floor, moving and shifting until you feel connected to the floor.

Now feel your back and bottom on the chair, sensing how the chair gives you support. Ask yourself if you are perching in the chair or allowing the chair to support you. Then try to settle in the chair more comfortably.

Adjust until you feel your comfort spot. Then take a few minutes to really enjoy the comfort of being supported by the chair and stabilized by the floor.

Take a look around and notice something that feels resourceful. For example, the tree right outside the window, a piece of art, the floor, a calming colour, and so on. Savor the resourceful feelings.

What do you notice now about your overall comfort (physically and emotionally)? Do you have the same feeling as when you started or somewhat different.

If you take your time with this exercise, you will be surprised at how much settling you can achieve in your nervous system in just a moment.

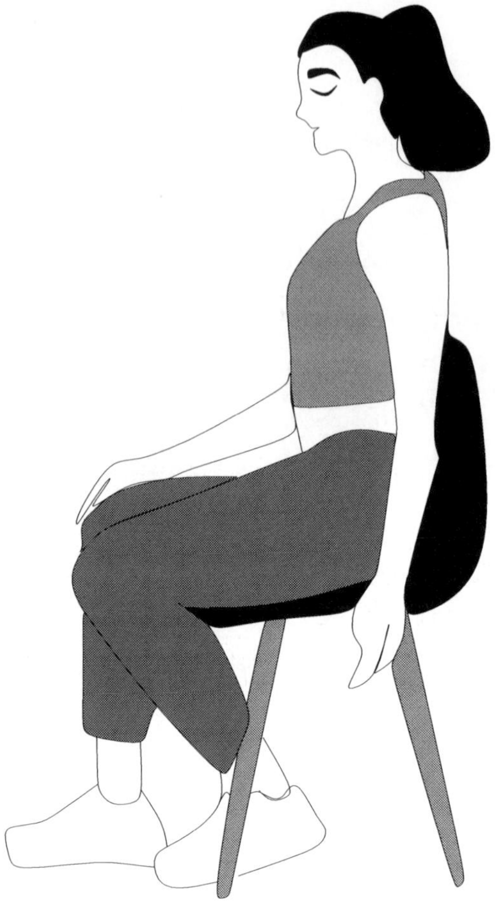

Long-Term Strategies for Sustained Healing

Any journey towards healing is not a sprint. Even if it is something as little as a bruise, you have to wash it so it doesn't get infected, clean it, and then cover it up for the body to heal itself. It takes your body a while for it to recover from surgery, so why do you want to heal from your trauma and anxiety in a few hours?

Healing is a marathon, it requires constant attention and consistency to achieve your desired result. I know sometimes, we feel like we've gotten to the root of the problem, but many times, we just have a simple understanding of the problem, and the road to healing remains.

Somatic therapy is a great way to address these problems and their causes, to sustain the healing you have achieved, you would need to be consistent in your exercises and activities. And you also need to be self-conscious about your healing.

In this section, we will explore some ways you can make conscious self-care an important part of your life and daily routine. What you are about to learn will help you build a strong foundation for your emotional well-being and help you consciously and consistently stay on track with your goals and aspirations.

Self-Care Practices for Sustained Healing

These are some somatic therapy practices and activities that you might be familiar with;

1. **Mindfulness:** This is a somatic practice that involves paying attention to your present moment and mindfully exploring your feelings without judgment. It gives you a chance to get out of your head, the thoughts, and worries that often trigger or increase your anxiety. Some benefits of mindfulness are;

   a. It helps to reduce stress and anxiety.

   b. It helps to improve your emotional regulation.

   c. It improves your self-awareness.

   d. It enhances your focus and concentration because you are now more self-aware and in the moment.

2. **Meditation:** This is a type of mindfulness. It involves focusing or concentrating on a particular object, sensation or thought and then fully exploring it without judgment. It has similar benefits to mindfulness. Here are some of the other benefits it has;

   a. It promotes relaxation and improves sleep quality.

   b. It improves emotional regulation and resilience.

3. **Yoga:** Yoga incorporates several somatic activities like breathing, body postures, and meditation. It makes you physically flexible and strong in addition to helping you stay mindful and calm. Its benefits include:

   a. Reduction of stress and anxiety.

   b. Improving the quality of your sleep.

   c. Improving your body awareness and coordination.

Now that we know some effective self-care practices, it is time to build your self-care toolkit.

Building a Self-Care Toolkit for Sustained Healing

The following are some tips to build your self-care toolkit;

1. **Identify your triggers:** what are some of the things that trigger your anxiety or trauma? It could be:

   a. A person
   b. A place
   c. A song
   d. A word
   e. A situation
   f. Food or drink.

Whatever your trigger is, write it down because this is the first step on this marathon of healing.

2. **Identify the physical sensations and emotions that accompany these triggers:** Do you feel tightness in your chest and anger or sadness? Write the physical sensations and emotions you experience when these triggers happen.

3. **Identify activities that help you cope with these triggers and sensations:** Recall the last time you felt any of these triggers, what or who helped you to get through it? Write it down. What are some other things you did that eased the pressure of these triggers? Write them down. Some proven coping mechanisms that you might want to try are;

    a. **Journaling:** it involves strategically putting down what you are going through, how it feels, how you want to feel, and what you need to do.

    b. **Physical activities:** things like exercising, yoga, running, and walking are great for relieving the pressure of your trauma and anxiety.

    c. **Breathing awareness:** this just involves you pausing from the frenzy around you to take note of how you are breathing; the texture, how long you can hold it, and if your belly or chest is rising. It is a great relaxation method.

    d. **Box breathing:** this involves a chain of breath that is of the same length. For example, you inhale for 2 seconds, hold your breath for 2 seconds, and finally exhale for 2 seconds. You can increase the time as you go.

e. **Seeking help:** for some people, their coping mechanism is speaking to a loved one. Whoever that is for you, add them to your toolkit. And if you don't have one, you can discover yours. Take an empty sheet and ask yourself, "Who are those who have helped me through this kind of difficult situation in the past?" Write down how they can help you now. You can add an extra portion where you write how you will reach out to them.

4. **Organize your toolkit:** when you are done with this. Organize it perfectly. Use the worksheet below as an example for a trigger.

Trigger

_____

_____

Physical Sensations	Emotions

Coping mechanisms that work for me.

_____

_____

_____

Coping mechanisms I want to try.

_____

_____

_____

Who can support me through this?

_____

How can I reach them?

Group Therapy and Components

Let's visualize this: Imagine a warm and welcoming place where you're not just meeting with your therapist but also connecting with people who are going through similar experiences. How would that feel? That's what group therapy offers. It's a space where, regardless of your progress, hearing others share their journeys can boost your confidence and reinforce your belief in healing.

Group therapy can be a very powerful tool in your journey to healing from anxiety and trauma. Let's take a look at some of the benefits of group therapy;

1. **Shared experiences:** Too many people are alone in their struggles with trauma and anxiety. Group therapy offers you an escape hatch for this by giving you people who understand your struggles because they lived or are living through the same thing. The atmosphere removes loneliness and isolation. And it also helps you with positive validation.

2. **Reduced or eliminated stigma:** There's a big stigma about going to therapy, and it can be hard for some people, but when you are with others with similar shared experiences, you can let your guard down and focus on your healing.

3. **Opportunities to learn from others:** Sometimes, there's a coping mechanism that works but you haven't discovered it yet. It could be a grounding mechanism or new information about

anything. Being in a room with people like you offers an opportunity to learn something that may help you later on.

4. **Support and encouragement:** Sometimes, all you want to do is quit and stop the lessons because of one thing or another. But being with people like you, who have the same experiences, you can support and encourage each other to continue.

Types of Group Therapy Approaches

1. **Support groups:** This is a group therapy that encourages sharing experiences and promoting support and encouragement.
2. **Psychoeducational groups:** It is similar to support groups but with something extra. It offers information and education on the reason for the group; it could be trauma and anxiety or it could be about substance abuse. The important thing here is that they offer education and support on these topics.
3. **Process groups:** Like the first two on this list, it offers education and support but it doesn't stop there, it goes deeper like helping you to explore the underlying physical and emotional effects of trauma and anxiety. This group encourages you to share your past experiences and helps you explore the impact it having on your life in the present moment.
4. **Skill-training groups:** This group offers support, encouragement, education, and most importantly, they equip you with the skills you need to manage your anxiety and trauma. One of the skills they help you learn is CBT (Cognitive-Behavioral Therapy).

Finding the most Suitable Group Therapy for Yourself

1. Consider the type you want.
2. Consider the size. How many people are you comfortable with in a group?
3. Consider the leader's qualifications and track record.
4. Consider how much time you have and how committed can you be.

These 4 things are important to consider when you are deciding to choose group therapy.

A Pathway to Easing Anxiety through Somatic Therapy

A large part of our lives as human beings involves solving problems. Many aspects of our lives require us to find solutions. For instance, when the heater refuses to work, you need to find a solution quickly. Or when you miss the last bus or train, your brain starts trying to find a way to get you home. When this happens, it is easy to feel anxious. Sometimes, the anxiety can set in before the situation even occurs.

Anxiety is a common part of our lives. We are often anxious about various things. However, when anxiety becomes prolonged, it can create problems that affect both our lives and the lives of those around us.

Your body is not just a tool for movement; it is much more than that. Have you ever noticed that when you are injured, you tend to be a bit cranky? Our bodies signal to us when something is amiss because they are connected to our minds. This connection is why your heart beats faster when you are startled and why you may struggle to speak when you are scared.

This mind-body connection is what somatic therapists refer to as the key to solving anxiety issues. Somatic therapy utilizes this connection, along with other exercises, to help us better connect with our bodies and minds.

Understanding this connection allows us to alleviate stress and anxiety more effectively.

Using Somatic Techniques to Soothe Anxiety

Somatic therapy employs several exercises that are important in easing your stress and anxiety, but it doesn't stop there, these exercises help you gain insights about who you are and how grew into the current version of yourself. Somatic therapy also helps you understand your body and it helps you identify the best coping mechanism for you.

Some of the exercises used in somatic therapy are;

- **Body Scan:** This exercise is based on the principle of the mind-body connection. It involves conducting a thorough mental scan of your entire body, from your head down to your toes. This exercise requires focused attention as you must take note of the physical sensations and emotions that arise during the scan. Finally, you are required to record this experience on paper.
- **Breath Work:** There are different types of breathing, but we are mostly exposed to one – the deep breathing technique. There are a few others like box breathing. In somatic therapy, these breathing techniques are called conscious breathing technique which is a somatic exercise itself.
- **Visualization:** This is a coping mechanism for stress and anxiety as it is for trauma. It involves focusing your mind and bringing something that soothes you into view. It could be a place, an object, or a person. Visualization is a soothing exercise, but it can be used to explore why you are anxious.

Somatic therapy involves exploration because that is the only way you can get to the root of what is causing your anxiety. You don't want to address the symptoms alone without touching the cause, because the symptoms will always reoccur if you don't address the root cause. That is why somatic therapy is about exploration and release. You explore until you find the cause and then release it.

Somatic Therapy Exercises and Grounding Techniques for Anxiety Relief

The following are some of the grounding techniques you can use when you feel anxious. Grounding techniques take you away from the scenario in your head making you anxious and it makes you stay present in the moment.

Some somatic grounding techniques you can use are;

1. **The 5 senses grounding or 5-4-3-2-1 technique.**

This grounding method requires you to engage all your senses.

You identify;

5 things you can see around you

4 things around you that you can touch

3 things you can hear

2 things you can smell around you

1 safe and edible thing you can taste

2. **The Rooting Visualization**

This is a grounding technique where you engage your imagination. It involves imagining roots extending from your feet with each breath you take. This method helps you visually imagine yourself standing solidly on the ground.

3. Weighted Objects

This object can be an object of comfort to you. It is always recommended to have one, you don't necessarily need to carry them around. It could be a ring, a ball, a pen. Etc. What matters is that whenever you touch it, you feel comfortable and relaxed.

There are two ways to do it;

- **The first one** involves your comfort object, weighted or not. It requires you to pick it up close your eyes and as you hold it, it is keeping you calm and in the present.
- **The second one** involves an actual weighted object. Take any type of stone or a weighted blanket. Feel its weight and check its solidity. Let it remind you that you are in the present.

These are just a few somatic therapy exercises you can use to ease your anxiety. Use the worksheet below to get a better understanding of how to use them to ease your anxiety.

Worksheet for Somatic Therapy and Anxiety

Exercise 1:

Body Scan

Instructions

- Get into a relaxed position, either sitting or lying down in a quiet part of your home.
- Close your eyes and take a few slow, deep breaths. Take note of your breath moving in and out.

Fill out this table chart, focusing on body sensations in each area.

Body Part	Sensations
Toes	

Feet & Ankles	
Calves & Knees	
Thighs & Hips	

Buttocks & Lower Back	
Stomach & Mid Back	
Chest & Upper Back	

Shoulders & Neck	
Arms & Hands	
Head	

How many body parts were tensed or tight? _____

Which sensation occurred the most?

_____

Briefly describe how the highest occurring sensation is associated with your anxiety.

_____

_____

_____

What emotions did you experience during the scan?

_____

_____

_____

_____

_____

How did your body feel before this exercise?

_____

_____

_____

How does your body feel now after this exercise?

_____

Exercise 2:

Grounding Techniques

5 Senses Grounding

Instructions:

Whenever you notice your anxiety creeping in, take a deep breath and look around you. Take note of your surroundings and engage your 5 senses.

Sight:

List 3 things you can see around you right now.

_____

_____

_____

Briefly describe each one.

1.

_____

_____

2.

_____

_____

3.

_____

_____

Hearing:

List 3 sounds you can hear right now.

_____

_____

_____

Briefly describe each one.

1.

_____

_____

2.

_____

_____

3.

_____

_____

What are you touching right now? Or what is safe around you that you can touch?

_____

Briefly describe its texture

_____

_____

Briefly describe its temperature

_____

_____

Briefly describe its pressure.

_____

_____

Smell:

Write 3 things you can smell right now.

_____

_____

_____

What is something you are eating/drinking or recently ate/drunk?

Briefly describe the texture

_____

_____

_____

Briefly describe the flavor.

_____

_____

_____

Briefly describe the taste.

_____

_____

How well did you feel grounded when you engaged your senses?

_____

_____

_____

_____

What emotions did you experience during this exercise?

_____

_____

_____

_____

How can you incorporate this exercise into your daily activities to help you cope with anxiety?

_____

_____

_____

_____

Box Breathing

- Sit or Stand comfortably.
- Inhale through your nose for 5 seconds. Do this through your nose.
- Hold this breath for 5 seconds
- Using your mouth as the outlet, exhale for 5 seconds.
- Repeat steps 2 to 4 up to 5 times.

How are you feeling before doing this exercise?

___

What triggered this feeling?

How did your body feel after this breathing exercise?

_____

_____

_____

How can you incorporate this breathing technique into your daily routine?

_____

_____

_____

_____

_____

Exercise 3:

Self-Care Plan

Identify your anxiety triggers. *Write 3 common anxiety triggers you have noticed.*

Trigger 1

_____

_____

_____

Trigger 2

_____

_____

_____

Trigger 3

_____

_____

Choose 1 grounding technique that you want to try from the two in exercise 2.

☐   5 Senses Grounding

☐   Box Breathing

How will you use this grounding technique for the triggers you wrote?

Trigger 1

_____

_____

Action Steps

_____

_____

_____

_____

_____

Trigger 2

_____

Action Steps

Trigger 3

Action Steps

What other self-care practices can you include in this plan?

SOMATIC THERAPY WORKBOOK

Section 1: Preparation

Part 1: Body Awareness Scan

Exercise 1: Body Mapping

Instructions

- Find a place in your home that is quiet and where you can't be disturbed.

- You can do this exercise by lying or sitting down, but make sure you are comfortable no matter your choice.

- Take deep breaths and close your eyes until you feel relaxed.

- Gently scan your body mentally. Start from your toes and keep scanning each part until you reach your head.

- Take note of which parts are uncomfortable, tensed, tight, or relaxed.

- When you are done scanning, get a blank sheet of paper, and outline your body on this paper.

- On this outline, mark the areas that are tensed, tight, and relaxed.

How did your body feel during this mental scan and mapping?

_____

_____

What surprises did you experience during this exercise?

What did you learn about yourself here?

What memories did you experience during this exercise? *Share one of them.*

_____

_____

_____

Which part of your body were you scanning when you remembered this memory?

_____

What emotions did you experience during this exercise? *Write the emotions and which body part you were scanning when you experienced it.*

_____

_____

_____

_____

Activity 1: Choose a time each day for you to practice this exercise.

Day	Time
Monday	

Tuesday	
Wednesday	
Thursday	
Friday	
Saturday	
Sunday	

Exercise 2: Sensory Exploration

- Find a place in your home that is quiet and where you can't be disturbed.

- You can do this exercise by lying down or sitting down, but make sure you are comfortable no matter what you choose.

- Take deep breaths and close your eyes until you feel relaxed.

- Now, let's explore your sensory experience.

Touch: Take note of how you and your skin feel when touched. Try with your hands and then some fabrics around you.

How does your body feel?

_____

_____

_____

Pressure: Pay attention to the points where your body touches the ground or the surface you are lying on.

How does it feel? What physical and emotional sensations do you notice?

_____

_____

_____

_____

Do you feel cool or warm? *Write your answer.*

_____

Hearing: What sounds can you hear as you are sitting or lying down?

_____

_____

_____

_____

Sight: With your eyes closed, what visual patterns can you observe?

What colors do you see/observe?

_____

_____

_____

What visual patterns did you observe? *Briefly describe this.*

_____

_____

_____

What sensations stood out during your exploration?

_____

_____

_____

What emotions or thoughts were associated with each sense?

Sensory	Thoughts/Emotions	Memories

Touch		
Pressure		

Sight		
Sound		

How did this exercise impact your overall well-being?

How did you feel before the exercise?	How did you feel after the exercise?

Activity 2: Choose a day and a time this week just to listen to your surroundings and then record your experience.

What day will you choose? _____

What time will you choose? _____

What did you hear during this activity?

_____

_____

_____

_____

_____

What thoughts or emotions arose during this activity?

_____

_____

_____

_____

_____

Exercise 3: Breath Observation

Instructions:

- Find a place in your home that is quiet and where you can't be disturbed.

- You can do this exercise by lying down or sitting down, but make sure you are comfortable no matter what you choose.

- Pay attention to every sensation you are feeling.

- Now, gently turn your attention towards your breath. Be careful so you don't alter it mistakenly.

- Pay attention to your breath. Don't try to take control, just focus on it. Is it shallow or deep, or is it fast or slow?

- Pay attention to your chest and stomach, take note of their rise and fall.

- Do this for 5 minutes, and if your mind wanders, gently shift your focus back to your breath.

What did you notice or learn about your breath?

_____

_____

_____

_____

_____

Did you observe any change in your breath during this exercise?

YES | NO

How did your breath change?

_____
_____
_____
_____

Were the changes linked with any thought or emotion?

YES | NO

What emotions caused a change in your breath?

_____
_____
_____
_____

How does your breath feel right now after this exercise?

_____

_____

_____

What did you learn about yourself after this exercise?

_____

_____

_____

Activity 3: Choose a convenient time every day to practice your breath observation.

What time is convenient for you every day? _____

This time take note of the physical sensations you feel as you are breathing.

What physical sensations did you experience?

_____

_____

_____

_____

Observe your breathing while you are on another task.

Which task will you observe your breath with? (E.g. running, walking, doing the dishes. etc.)

Briefly describe your breathing during this task.

Part 2: Grounding Techniques

Exercise 4: Earth Connection

Instructions:

- This exercise will be done outdoors. So find a comfortable outdoor location with natural ground where it is safe to stand barefooted.
- If you can't stay outdoors, you can stand barefooted on solid ground in your home.
- Take a few moments for your body to settle, stretch your body, and take note of the sensations you feel.
- Breathe in and imagine your breath flowing through your body, down to your legs, and into the ground.
- Visualize your breaths like roots extending out of your feet and securing you to the ground.
- Take more deep breaths and feel this support from the earth.
- Take note of how your body feels and how your posture changes.

Briefly describe how your body feels when you connected with the earth.

_____

_____

Did your body or posture change during this exercise?

YES | NO

Briefly describe how your posture changed.

_____

_____

_____

_____

What thoughts or emotions did you notice while connecting to the earth?

_____

_____

_____

_____

Briefly describe how your body feels now that you have completed this exercise.

_____

_____

_____

_____

Recall a time you felt this kind of support and grounding in your life.

Briefly describe the situation.

_____

_____

_____

_____

Briefly describe how it makes you feel.

_____

_____

_____

Exercise 5: Sensory Anchoring

Instructions

- Find a place in your home that is quiet and where you can't be disturbed.

- You can do this exercise by lying down or sitting down, but make sure you are comfortable no matter what you choose.

- Give your body enough time to settle, while you wait, take deep breaths slowly until you feel settled.

- Pay attention to all the sensations you are feeling. It could be the sensation of how your breath enters and leaves your nose or how your clothes are touching your body.

- Now, gently shift awareness to your senses.

Sight

Choose one object in your view.

What is this object? *Briefly describe this object.*

_____

_____

_____

What color is this object?

_____

What texture does it have?

_____

How will you describe its shape?

_____

_____

What other details can you notice?

_____

_____

Sound

Focus on your surroundings. Take note of the sounds you hear. Choose one of these sounds.

How loud is this sound?

_____

How will you rate its quality? ☐ Great ☐ Good ☒ Okay

Does it have a special rhythm?   YES | NO

Briefly describe this rhythm.

_____

_____

_____

Smell

Focus on your surroundings, but pay attention to the scents around you.

Do you notice any pleasant scent around you?　　　　YES | NO

If yes, can you bring this scent closer?　　　YES | NO

If yes, do it. If no, recall a recent pleasant and calming scent you experienced recently.

Briefly describe this scent.

_____

_____

Briefly describe the effect this scent has on you.

_____

_____

_____

Taste

Do you have any edible food substance around you?

YES | NO

If yes, eat it.

What is this edible food?

_____

Briefly describe its taste.

_____

_____

_____

How does this food substance make you feel?

_____

_____

_____

If your answer is no, recall the last thing you ate. *What was it?*

Briefly describe the taste.

How does it make you feel?

Touch

Recall the last time you felt a pleasant sensation on your skin. *What happened? Briefly describe what you felt.*

Briefly describe how it made you feel.

_____

_____

_____

Read the statements below and tick the one that resonates with you.

☐ I experienced a feeling of calmness as I focused on my senses.

☐ Visualizing these senses helped me stay in the present.

☐ The sensory details I experienced became vivid.

Which sense was easy for you to anchor?

_____

Why was it easy for you?

_____

_____

_____

How did this exercise impact your emotional state and your body?

_____

_____

_____

_____

_____

How can you integrate this exercise into your daily routine?

_____

_____

_____

_____

_____

Exercise 6: Mindful Walking

Instructions

- Identify a comfortable place where you can walk. It can either be indoor or outdoor.

- You want to stay relaxed. Take note of your breath and air is going in and coming out. Also, take note of what you feel as your feet touch the ground.

- Start walking slowly and deliberately, but while you do this pay attention to the physical sensations you experience with each step you take.

- Pay attention to what you feel when you move and how your chest moves up and down.

- Engage all your senses as you move, take note of what you see, what you hear, feel on your skin, and what you can smell. Just observe everything you see and feel, don't judge.

- Your mind could wander, don't fret, and gently bring awareness back to your walk and your breath.

- Engage this exercise for about 10 minutes.

Where did you choose for your walk?

☐ Indoor

☐ Outdoor

Briefly describe some of the things you noticed in your body during this mindful walk.

_____

_____

_____

What do you think your senses contributed to this experience?

_____

_____

_____

_____

Did your mind wander?   YES | NO

If yes, what do you think distracted you?

_____

_____

_____

Where did your mind go and why do you think it went there?

_____

_____

_____

How did you bring your attention and awareness back to the present?

_____

_____

_____

How did you feel before the mindful walk?

_____

_____

How did you feel after the mindful walk?

_____

_____

_____

How can you integrate mindful walking into your daily activities? *Briefly describe how you will do this.*

_____

_____

_____

_____

What regular daily activity will you pair your mindful walking with?

_____

Activity 4: Choose a day this week where you will engage in mindful working for about 30 minutes.

Which day did you choose? _____

What time will you engage in this exercise? _____

Where is a quiet, safe, and comfortable place to do it?

_____

How will you stay accountable?

_____

_____

Part 3: Breathe Awareness

Exercise 7: Your Personal Sanctuary

Instructions

- Find a place in your home that is quiet and where you can't be disturbed.

- You can do this exercise by lying down or sitting down, but make sure you are comfortable no matter what you choose.

- Give your body enough time to settle, while you wait, take deep breaths slowly until you feel settled.

- Imagine you are entering a place that is peaceful or safe. This place could be a real-life place or it could be imagined.

- Make use of your senses to visualize this place better. Take note of what you see, hear, smell, taste, and feel.

- Take note of everything in this safe place: the plants and animals.

- Pay attention to how your body feels in this place.

Briefly describe your imaginary sanctuary.

_____

_____

_____

_____

Write 3 things you can see in your sanctuary.

_____

_____

_____

Write one significant smell in your sanctuary.

_____

Write one significant thing you taste in this sanctuary.

_____

Write 3 things you can hear in this sanctuary.

_____

_____

_____

Briefly describe how you felt in your sanctuary.

_____

_____

How can your special sanctuary help you?

_____

_____

_____

_____

_____

Activity 5: Draw or Record a description of your sanctuary.

Instructions

- Take a large sheet of paper and then sketch your safe space.
- Use different pencil and pen colors to make your work stand out.
- Take a recorder or you can use the one on your phone.
- Record a description of what your sanctuary looks like.
- Take note of the physical features you can see, the smells you can smell, how the air feels, what you can taste, and the plants, animals, and other objects in your sanctuary.

Choose a day to visualize this sanctuary this week.

Day _____

Time _____

Choose how you want to record your experience

☐ Drawing

☐ Voice Recording

Briefly describe how you felt with this exercise today.

_____

_____

_____

Exercise 8: Discover Your Emotional Guardians

Recall a time you experienced a strong emotion. Briefly describe what happened.

_____

_____

_____

Which emotion did you experience?

☐ Anger

☐ Sadness

☐ Fear

☐ Joy

☐ Others

_____

_____

_____

What physical sensation did you experience with this emotion?

_____

_____

What part of you do you think is protecting you from feeling this emotion?

Briefly describe this emotional guidance.

What message do you think this guidance is trying to tell you?

_____

_____

_____

How can you be more compassionate towards your emotions and your emotional guidance?

_____

_____

_____

_____

_____

Activity 6: Have a friendly chat with your emotional guidance.

Once you've identified your emotional guidance, have a dialogue with this character.

Recall the emotion you got from that situation. Ask your guidance why it's protecting you from this emotion. Sit and listen.

_____

_____

_____

_____

How can you reassure your guidance?

_____

_____

_____

_____

Exercise 9: Anchoring Objects

Recall a time you were distressed with a strong emotion. *What happened?*

_____

_____

What emotions did you experience?

_____

_____

_____

_____

What are some objects that hold special meaning for you?

_____

_____

_____

_____

Choose one of these objects to explore.

Which one did you choose?

_____

Briefly describe this object.

What material is it made from?

_____

_____

Describe its shape and size.

_____

_____

_____

Why is this object meaningful to you?

_____

_____

_____

_____

Imagine you are holding your anchoring object. *What sensations do you notice?*

_____

_____

_____

_____

_____

How do you plan to use your anchoring object throughout the day?

_____

_____

_____

_____

What are some challenges you might face in using your anchoring object?

_____

_____

_____

_____

What are some other objects you can use as your anchoring objects?

Section 2: Exploration

Part 1: Body Mapping and Tracking

Exercise 10: Sensation Exploration

Take time to explore your sensations and record them.

Instructions:

- Choose a day to practice some somatic therapy exercises.
- Do a body scan and record your experience.

What day did you choose? _____

Choose a time. _____

What physical sensations did you experience after your scan? Use the table below to log these sensations and where you felt them on your body.

Sensations	Where you felt them.

How did these sensations change before and after this scan?

How did you feel before the scan?

_____

_____

_____

_____

How did you feel after the scan?

_____

_____

_____

_____

What changed?

_____

_____

_____

What emotions did you experience during this scan?

_____

_____

_____

_____

How are these emotions connected to your physical sensations?

Exercise 11: Emotional Body Scan

Instructions;

Find a comfortable place in your home to sit or lie down in silence.

Sit or lie down comfortably and close your eyes.

- Take slow and deep breaths till you feel settled.

- When you feel calm, scan your body, from the head to the toe. Take note of the physical sensations you are feeling. It could be warmth, cold, tension, or relaxation.

- Pay attention to areas with the most tension/discomfort and the emotions that arise.

- Observe these emotions for about 5 minutes without judgment.

- Record your experience.

Body Part	Physical Sensation	Associated Emotions
Head & Neck		
Shoulders & Upper Back		

Chest & Abdomen		
Lower Back & Hips		

Arms & Hands		
Leg & Feet		

What were the most noticeable sensations you experience?

_____

_____

_____

_____

What significant insight did you gain from this exercise?

_____

_____

_____

What change did you notice in your emotional state during this scan?

_____

_____

_____

_____

Which areas of your body surprised you?

_____

_____

_____

_____

How can you use this exercise to detect and manage your emotions in the future?

_____

_____

_____

_____

Exercise 12: Trauma Release Movement

Instructions:

- Wear clothes comfortable for movement.
- Find a safe and open space where you can move freely.
- Take deep breaths to settle yourself, and then carefully feel your feet planted on the floor.
- Start your movement by swaying side-to-side.
- Explore some other different types of movements.
- Pay attention to sensations such as tightness and uncomfortable areas.
- Acknowledge emotions that come up and let your body express these emotions through your movement.
- Keep moving for about 10.

What movements did you explore? Tick the one that applies.

☐ Stretching

☐ Jumping

☐ Shaking

☐ Others

_____

_____

Where did you feel tightness in your body?

☐ Shoulder

☐ Head

☐ Neck

☐ Toes

☐ Belly

☐ Hands

☐ Others

What emotions did you experience?

☐ Anger

☐ Sadness

☐ Fear

☐ Joy

☐ Others

Briefly describe the emotional changes that you experienced.

Were you hesitant to move in the beginning?   YES | NO

Briefly describe why you choose your answer above.

Remember when you were expressing your emotions through movements? Which emotions were harder to express.

Choose one of the emotions above. *What emotion did you choose?*

What memory does it remind you of? Briefly describe this memory.

How has this emotion affected you in the past?

How does it affect you now?

Activity 7: Choose one movement you want to use to release this emotion this week.

Which movement will you use? _____

What day will you engage in this movement? _____

How many times will you use this movement this week? _____

What days will practice this movement?
_____

Log how you felt before and how you felt after the practice.

How did you feel before this activity?

_____

_____

_____

How did you feel after this activity?

_____

_____

_____

Part 2: Emotional Release Techniques

Exercise 13: Cathartic Writing

Instructions

- Find a place in your home that is quiet and where you can't be disturbed.

- Get writing materials and take deep breaths until you feel relaxed.

- Write a letter to yourself. Choose from the prompts below.

- Write and let it flow. Don't judge and don't worry about grammar or spelling mistakes.

- Set a timer for yourself and as you are writing pay attention to the physical sensations and emotions you experience.

- When the timer goes off or when you are done writing. Take deep breaths before you record your experience.

Writing prompts

Choose the letter you want to write.

☐ A letter to this difficult emotion. *Write the emotion.* _____

☐ A writing about a part of you. *Describe what it is and how it makes you feel.*

☐ A writing about if your body could talk.

Which prompt did you choose?

_____

_____

Why did you choose it?

_____

_____

_____

Write here

What emotions came up as you were writing?

_____
_____
_____
_____

What physical sensations did you experience as you were writing?

_____
_____
_____
_____

What shifts did you notice?

_____
_____
_____
_____

What part of this exercise was more challenging?

_____

_____

_____

How can you use this exercise for your emotional care in the future?

_____

_____

_____

_____

Exercise 14: Expressing Emotions through Art

- Find a place in your home that is quiet and where you can't be disturbed.

- Make sure you are comfortable no matter your choice.

- Take deep breaths and choose an emotion you want to express artistically.

- Let this emotion fill you. Gently explore this emotion without judgment.

- Pay attention to how you feel, especially your physical sensations.

- Move and let your mind guide your art.

Choose the emotion you want to express

☐ Anger

☐ Sadness

☐ Fear

☐ Joy

☐ Frustration

☐ Confusion

☐ Other (Write it below)

_____

_____

What emotion did you choose?

Why did you choose this emotion?

What materials did you use for your art expression?

What images, colors, or thoughts come to your mind?

_____

_____

_____

What physical sensations can you notice?

_____

_____

_____

_____

What new knowledge or insights did you learn about yourself during this exercise?

_____

_____

_____

_____

_____

How can you use this exercise in the future to manage emotions?

_____

_____

_____

Part 3: Exploring Trauma Timeline

Exercise 15: Lifeline Drawing

Instructions:

Find a place in your house that is comfortable, silent, and free of disturbance.

- Settle yourself and feel present in the moment.
- Now imagine your life is a straight line starting from the left (birth) and running to the right (present moment).
- Draw this line and you can either draw it up to represent high times in your life or draw the line down to represent low times in your life.
- Take your time to feel the emotions and sensations associated with these events in your life.
- When you are done drawing, pause, and observe your lifeline.

Choose 3 high points in your lifeline and then identify the emotions and sensations associated with them.

High Points	Emotions	Physical Sensations

1.

2.

3.

Choose 3 low points in your lifeline and then identify the emotions and sensations associated with them.

Low Points	Emotions	Physical Sensations
1.		
2.		
3.		

What patterns did you notice in your lifeline?

_____

_____

_____

_____

What did this lifeline reveal to you about you and your life?

_____

_____

_____

_____

What is something that surprised you in this exercise?

_____

_____

What emotions did you experience while creating this lifeline?

_____

_____

_____

_____

How do you think doing this exercise can help you in the future?

_____

_____

_____

_____

What does your timeline tell you about your strength and resilience?

_____

_____

_____

_____

Exercise 16: Sensation Reflection

Instructions:

- Take a few moments throughout your day, pause for a few minutes, and check in with yourself and your body.

- Take note of the physical sensations you experience.

What time did you check in with your body?

_____

How many times did you check in?

_____

Highlight the physical sensations you experienced, where you felt them, and their intensity.

Physical Sensation	Location in the Body	Intensity %

What patterns did you notice throughout the day?

_____

_____

_____

_____

What emotions were associated with certain physical sensations?

_____

_____

_____

How can this body awareness help you understand your emotions in order to navigate your day better?

_____

_____

_____

_____

Exercise 17: Compassionate Self-Reflection

Instructions:

- Find a place in your home that is quiet and where you can't be disturbed.

- You can do this exercise by lying or sitting down, but make sure you are comfortable no matter your choice.

- Settle yourself with deep breaths and then take note of all the sensations and emotions flooding your body.

- Recall a recent situation that triggered a difficult emotion.

What emotion did you experience?

_____

_____

Briefly describe the situation that triggered this emotion.

_____

_____

_____

What physical sensations did you experience?

_____

_____

_____

Imagine you are sitting with a friend going through the same thing.
What compassionate thing will you say to them?

_____

_____

_____

_____

Now, personalize and repeat this to yourself.

Exercise 18: Self-Compassion Body Scan

Instructions:

- Sit still or lie down and perform a body scan. Pay attention to the physical sensations and emotions that arise.
- Once you discover a tight or tense area, place a hand on this part, take deep breaths, and imagine each breath sending warmth and relaxing energy to this point.

What physical sensations did you experience during this scan? *Write 3*

_____

_____

_____

What emotions did you experience? *Write 3.*

_____

_____

_____

How did this self-compassion exercise help you release tension?

_____

_____

How can this exercise help you in the future?

Section 3: Healing Tools

Part 1: Self Holding and Compassion

Exercise 19: Heart Hug

Instructions:

- Find a place in your home that is quiet and where you can't be disturbed.
- Sit straight or stand upright.
- Take deep breaths to settle and let your body relax.
- Give yourself a big bear hug with your eyes closed.
- Gently squeeze yourself in a hug with comfortable pressure.
- Breathe deeply and feel your body soften.

Briefly describe how this hug felt.

_____

_____

_____

What emotions arise during this exercise?

_____

_____

_____

_____

What did this exercise reveal to you about the need for self-compassion?

_____

_____

_____

How can you incorporate this self-care exercise into your daily routine?

_____

_____

_____

_____

Exercise 20: Loving-Kindness Meditation

Instructions:

- Find a comfortable and quiet place.
- Close your eyes and breathe deeply a few times.
- Imagine a gentle white light of love surrounding you.
- Silently repeat kind phrases to yourself. Continue until you feel good.
- Send this kindness to someone you care about. Also, imagine them surrounded by the white light and repeat kind phrases for them.

What kind words/phrases did you say to yourself?

_____

_____

_____

_____

_____

Why did you choose these phrases?

_____

_____

Did you experience a feeling of well-being after this exercise?

YES | NO

Briefly describe your experience and feelings of well-being if your answer is yes.

_____

_____

_____

_____

Who did you send kindness to? *Write their name.*

_____

What kind phrase/word did you use for this person?

_____

_____

_____

Exercise 21: Mirror Affirmations

Instructions:

- Find a quiet space in your house that has a mirror. Breathe deeply and allow your body to settle in.

- Look in the mirror.

- Say a simple affirmation (e.g., "I am worthy"). Take note of how your body responds. Do this for a few minutes.

- After a few minutes, choose a different affirmation that resonates with you. Repeat this affirmation and continue looking kindly at yourself kindly in the mirror.

- Continue for 5-10 minutes, experimenting with different affirmations.

What affirmation did you start with?

_____
_____

Briefly explain your choice with this affirmation. *Why did you choose it?*

_____
_____
_____

What physical sensations did you notice as you said the first affirmation?

_____

_____

_____

_____

_____

Which affirmation resonated with you the most from the ones you used?

_____

_____

Did you experience any emotional shift as you repeated these affirmations?

YES | NO

If yes, what emotional shift did you experience?

_____

_____

_____

_____

Did you notice any negative thoughts arise? YES | NO

What negative thoughts arose? *Write 3.*

_____

_____

_____

How did you feel when you noticed these negative thoughts?

_____

_____

_____

How did you bring awareness back to your affirmations?

_____

_____

_____

Briefly describe your overall experience with this exercise.

_____

_____

_____

Part 2: Progressive Muscle Relaxation

Exercise 22: Body Scan with Progressive Muscle Relaxation

Instructions:

- Find a place in your home that is quiet and where you can't be disturbed.
- You can do this exercise by lying or sitting down, but make sure you are comfortable no matter your choice.
- Take deep breaths and close your eyes until you feel relaxed.
- Carefully scan your body from your toes to your head.
- Notice any sensations without judgment.
- Carefully tense the muscles on the table below for 5 seconds each. Then relax them for 10 seconds. Record the physical sensations you feel.

Muscle Group	Physical Sensation
Toes	

Calves	
Thighs	
Buttocks	
Abdomen	
Chest	
Back	

Shoulders	
Arms & Hands	
Face & Neck	

Which parts were tense?

_____
_____
_____
_____

What emotions were common with these tense areas?

_____
_____

_____

_____

_____

How did your body feel after completing the body scan + PMR?

_____

_____

_____

What did this exercise teach you about yourself?

_____

_____

_____

_____

_____

Exercise 23: Guided Progressive Muscle Relaxation Script

Instructions:

- Follow the table below to follow the guided progressive muscle relaxation exercise.
- Follow the prompt in the first column. Then tick what you feel (tight/tense or relaxed). Finally, write any other thing you feel.

Muscle Group	Tensed	Relaxed	Notes
Forehead: raise your eyebrows.			
Eyes: squint till they are completely shut.			

Jaw: Clench your teeth.			
Neck: Press your neck hard.			
Shoulders: Shrug your shoulders.			

Upper back: Arch your upper back.			
Chest: Suck your stomach in.			
Stomach: Tighten their muscles.			

Lower back: press your back into the chair or floor.			
Buttocks: Clench the muscles.			
Thighs: Squeeze both legs together.			

Calves: Point your toes.			
Feet: Curl your toes.			

Focus on your overall feeling. What parts are tense?

_____

_____

_____

_____

Revisit these areas. Tense and release them again. Repeat this for about 5 minutes.

Briefly describe the state of your body before the exercise. *How was it?*

_____

_____

_____

Which areas are more tense than others? *Write 3.*

_____

_____

_____

Briefly describe the state of your body after the exercise.

_____

_____

_____

How can you incorporate this exercise into your daily activity for managing stress?

_____

Part 3: Somatic Yoga Sequences

Exercise 24: Grounding Flow

Instructions:

- Find a quiet space in your house and wear comfortable clothes.
- Stand upright and place your feet hip-width apart.
- Follow the prompts.

Neck Rolls:

- Gently roll your head. Go in circles.

Do you feel any tension melt away in your neck and shoulders?

YES | NO

Briefly describe how it feels.

_____

_____

_____

Arm Circles:

- Loosen up your shoulders.
- Make small circles with your arms, and go forward and back.

- Feel your shoulder blades move and any tightness ease up.

Did you feel it?   YES | NO

Spinal Twists:

- With your feet still hip-width apart, gently twist your torso from side to side.

- Keep your hips facing forward.

- Notice how your spine is moving and any areas of your body that feel restricted.

Is a part of your body restricted?   YES | NO

Which part is it?

_____

_____

How does it affect your body?

_____

_____

_____

How did your body feel throughout these sequences?

_____

_____

_____

_____

What areas of tension or tightness did you notice?

_____

_____

_____

How did your breath change during these movements?

_____

_____

_____

How do you feel after this exercise?

_____

_____

_____

Section 4: Integration

Part 1: Daily Routine

Exercise 25: Morning Somatic Check-In

Instructions:

- Find a place in your home that is quiet and where you can't be disturbed.

- Close your eyes and sit or lie down quietly for a few minutes.

- Take a few deep breaths and settle in. Notice your breath moving.

- Do a quick body scan. Use the table below.

Morning Somatic Check-In

Body Part	Physical Sensations	Intensity
	(*Circle the sensation you are feeling*). *If you don't see any tension, leave it blank.*	(*rate the intensity over 5. 5 being the highest*).

Head & Neck	Pressure Tension Headache	
Shoulders & Upper Back	Pressure Tension	
Chest & Abdomen	Tightness Heaviness Fluttering	
Lower Back & Hips	Aches Stiffness Discomfort	

Arms & Hands	Tension	
	Weakness	
	Tingling	
Legs & Feet	Heaviness	
	Coldness	
	Discomfort	

What is your overall % energy this morning? _____

Why do you think that is your energy level?

_____

_____

What emotions did you wake up to this morning?

_____

_____

_____

Why do you think you woke up with this emotion?

_____

_____

_____

Choose one emotion to explore. Which one did you choose?

_____

Why did you choose it?

_____

_____

Is it related to an unresolved situation?   YES | NO

What situation is it related to? *Briefly describe this situation.*

_____

_____

_____

What can you do to resolve this emotion?

_____

_____

_____

_____

Exercise 26: Somatic Breaks

Instructions:

- Set time for somatic breaks.
- Do simple somatic exercises you have learned in this book.

Set a time and interval that works for you. *What time did you choose?*
_____

What interval did you choose? _____

Pause when the timer stops and do a quick scan.

What physical sensations did you notice?

_____

_____

_____

_____

If you can, stand up and do simple stretching exercises. Make sure you are taking deep breaths.

Take a moment to ground yourself.

Use the 5 senses grounding method. Take a clean sheet of paper.

Write 1 thing you can taste.

_____

Write 2 things you can smell.

_____

_____

Write 3 you can hear.

_____

_____

_____

Write 4 things you can touch.

_____

_____

_____

_____

_____

Write 5 things you can see.

_____

_____

_____

_____

_____

Set an intention before you go back to your regular activity.

What is your intention for the next interval before your break?

_____

_____

_____

How did regular somatic breaks impact your stress levels today?

_____

_____

_____

_____

What physical sensations did I experience the most today?

_____

_____

_____

_____

What movements were the most helpful today?

_____

_____

_____

_____

How can I make somatic breaks a regular part of my daily activities?

_____

_____

_____

_____

_____

Exercise 27: Evening Reflection

Instructions:

- Close your eyes, take deep breaths, and let your body settle in for a quiet moment.

- Check-in with your body: take note of any tightness, relaxation, or warmth.

- Take note of your emotions as well. Are you calm, stressed, happy? Don't judge.

- Briefly recall and think about your day. What highs and lows did you experience, and how did you handle them?

What physical sensations did you experience today and where did you experience them?

_____

_____

_____

_____

_____

What emotions did you experience today?

_____

_____

_____

What were the important highlights of your day? *What highs did you experience?*

_____

_____

_____

_____

_____

What lows did you experience?

_____

_____

_____

_____

_____

What challenges did you experience?

_____

_____

_____

How did you resolve these challenges? *What coping strategies did you use?*

_____

_____

_____

_____

_____

What did you learn from your body awareness today?

What intention do you have for tomorrow?

What do you want to focus on?

What do you want to let go of?

Part 2: Reflective Journaling

Exercise 28: Triggers and Responses

Instructions:

- Briefly describe a recent situation that triggered an emotional response: who, what, where, when did it go down?

Who was there?

_____

_____

_____

Briefly describe what happened.

_____

_____

_____

When did it happen?

_____

_____

What emotional response was triggered?

_____

_____

What physical sensations did you notice?

_____

_____

_____

_____

How would you have responded to this trigger in the past?

_____

_____

_____

How has this response impacted you in the past?

_____

_____

How will you respond if it happens now?

What did you learn about your triggers and responses?

How did your body communicate triggers and their impact?

What healthy copy mechanism can you learn to help you manage your triggers in the future?

_____

_____

_____

_____

How can you be self-compassionate when trying to manage your triggers?

_____

_____

_____

_____

Exercise 29: Future Intentions

Instructions:

- Get comfortable and then take a few deep breaths to settle in.
- Close your eyes and imagine yourself in the future – thriving, living your best life. Focus on the positive feelings in your body.

How does your body feel in the future?

☐ Strong

☐ Energized

☐ Relaxed

Write down 3 intentions for your future that light you up.

_____

_____

_____

Exercise 30: Gratitude

Instructions:

- Get comfortable and take a few breaths to settle in.
- Think of something (or someone) awesome in your life. Big or small, it doesn't matter.
- Close your eyes and feel the gratitude in your body.
- Notice that feeling for a few moments. Open your eyes.

Who is this awesome person in your life?

_____

What makes them awesome?

_____

_____

_____

What is something you are grateful for in your life?

_____

_____

Why are you grateful for this thing?

_____

_____

_____

_____

_____

What physical sensations do you notice when you think about this amazing thing and person?

_____

_____

_____

_____

_____

How can you cultivate this feeling of gratitude throughout your day?

_____

_____

28-day exercise plan

Day	Morning	Afternoon	Evening
1	Grounding (5 mins)	Diaphragmatic Breathing (10 mins)	Progressive Muscle Relaxation (20 mins)
2	Self-regulation (Journaling)	Somatic Yoga (20 mins)	The Voo Breath (5 mins)
3	Resourcing and Visualization (15 mins)	Shake Out the Tension (5 mins)	Walking Meditation (15 mins)
4	Grounding (5 mins)	Sensory Awareness (10 mins)	Felt Sense (10 mins)
5	Self-regulation (Affirmations)	Heel Drops (5 mins)	Recalling a Kindness (10 mins)
6	Resourcing and Visualization (15 mins)	Body Mapping (20 mins)	Self-Holding (5 mins)
7	Grounding (5 mins)	Orienting (5 mins)	Closed Loop Connection to Your Body (10 mins)
8	Self-regulation (Mindful Breathing)	Wave Breathing (10 mins)	Pendulation (5 mins)
9	Resourcing and Visualization (15 mins)	Containment With Safe Touch (10 mins)	Rhythmic Movement (10 mins)
10	Grounding (5 mins)	Body Movement Technique (15 mins)	Bioenergy (10 mins)
11	Self-regulation (Gratitude List)	Butterfly Hug (5 mins)	Goddess Pose (10 mins)
12	Resourcing and Visualization (15 mins)	Wipe Away (5 mins)	Shaking (5 mins)
13	Grounding (5 mins)	When You Felt Most Like Yourself (Reflection)	Notice Your Current Physical Comfort (5 mins)

14	Self-regulation (Guided Imagery)	Somatic Yoga (20 mins)	The Voo Breath (5 mins)
15	Resourcing and Visualization (15 mins)	Shake Out the Tension (5 mins)	Walking Meditation (15 mins)
16	Grounding (5 mins)	Sensory Awareness (10 mins)	Felt Sense (10 mins)
17	Self-regulation (Affirmations)	Heel Drops (5 mins)	Recalling a Kindness (10 mins)
18	Resourcing and Visualization (15 mins)	Body Mapping (20 mins)	Self-Holding (5 mins)
19	Grounding (5 mins)	Orienting (5 mins)	Closed Loop Connection to Your Body (10 mins)
20	Self-regulation (Mindful Breathing)	Wave Breathing (10 mins)	Pendulation (5 mins)
21	Resourcing and Visualization (15 mins)	Containment With Safe Touch (10 mins)	Rhythmic Movement (10 mins)
22	Grounding (5 mins)	Body Movement Technique (15 mins)	Bioenergy (10 mins)
23	Self-regulation (Gratitude List)	Butterfly Hug (5 mins)	Goddess Pose (10 mins)
24	Resourcing and Visualization (15 mins)	Wipe Away (5 mins)	Shaking (5 mins)
25	Grounding (5 mins)	When You Felt Most Like Yourself (Reflection)	Notice Your Current Physical Comfort (5 mins)
26	Self-regulation (Choose your preferred method)	Diaphragmatic Breathing (10 mins)	Progressive Muscle Relaxation (20 mins)
27	Review and Reflect on the past weeks	Choose 2-3 favorite exercises to practice	Freeform Movement and Creative Expression
28	Grounding (5 mins)	Setting Intentions for Future Practice	Choose 1 self-care activity to prioritize

Important Notes:

- **Customization:** Feel free to adjust this plan to suit your individual needs and preferences. Some exercises may resonate more with you than others.

- **Guidance:** If you're new to these techniques, seek guidance from a therapist or trauma-informed practitioner. They can offer personalized instructions and support.

- **Listen to Your Body:** Pay attention to how your body responds to each exercise and do not hesitate to tweak any exercise that makes you feel uneasy.

This plan is a starting point. As you progress, you can experiment with different techniques and create a routine that best supports your healing journey.

The Trauma-Healing Diet

Key Principles:

- **Whole Foods:** Focus on unprocessed foods like veggies, fruits, lean proteins, whole grains, and healthy fats.
- **Gut Health:** Support your gut microbiome with fermented foods and fiber.
- **Hydration:** Water is very good for the body, drink more of water to fill your day.
- **Anti-inflammatory:** Include foods rich in antioxidants and omega-3 fatty acids.
- **Blood Sugar Balance:** Choose complex carbohydrates and limit added sugar.

Daily Meal Template:

- **Breakfast:**
  - Option 1: Oatmeal (½ cup dry oats) with berries (½ cup) and nuts/seeds (1 tbsp).
  - Option 2: Greek yogurt (1 cup) with fruit (½ cup) and granola (¼ cup).
  - Option 3: Eggs (2) scrambled with vegetables (½ cup) and whole-wheat toast (1 slice).
- **Lunch:**
  - Option 1: Salad with mixed greens (2 cups), protein (4 oz cooked chicken/fish/tofu), vegetables (1 cup), and a vinaigrette dressing (2 tbsp).

- o Option 2: Soup (1 bowl) and a whole-wheat sandwich (2 slices bread) with lean protein and vegetables.
- o Option 3: Leftovers from dinner.
- **Dinner:**
  - o Option 1: Baked salmon (4 oz) with roasted vegetables (1 cup) and brown rice (½ cup cooked).
  - o Option 2: Lentil soup (1 bowl) with whole-wheat bread (1 slice) and a side salad.
  - o Option 3: Stir-fry with tofu/chicken/beef (4 oz), vegetables (2 cups), and brown rice/quinoa (½ cup cooked).
- **Snacks (2-3 per day):**
  - o Fruits (apple, banana, berries)
  - o Vegetables (carrot sticks, celery, cucumber)
  - o Nuts/seeds (almonds, walnuts, pumpkin seeds)
  - o Yogurt (plain or Greek)
  - o Hard-boiled eggs

Day	Breakfast	Lunch	Dinner
1	Oatmeal with berries & nuts	Salad with chicken, mixed greens, avocado, and vinaigrette	Baked salmon with roasted broccoli and brown rice
2	Greek yogurt with fruit (banana, blueberries) & granola	Lentil soup with whole-wheat bread & side salad (mixed greens, cucumber, tomato)	Stir-fry with tofu, broccoli, carrots, and brown rice
3	Eggs (2) scrambled with spinach and whole-wheat toast	Leftovers from dinner (stir-fry)	Salad with grilled chicken or fish,

			quinoa, and a lemon-tahini dressing
4	Oatmeal with sliced apple, cinnamon, and walnuts	Turkey or veggie burger on whole-wheat bun with avocado and a side salad	Baked chicken breast with roasted sweet potatoes and green beans
5	Greek yogurt with mixed berries and a sprinkle of chia seeds	Leftovers from dinner (baked chicken)	Lentil stew with brown rice and a side of steamed kale
6	Smoothie (banana, spinach, almond milk, protein powder)	Salad with black beans, corn, bell peppers, avocado, and a lime-cilantro dressing	Stir-fry with shrimp, snap peas, broccoli, and brown rice
7	Oatmeal with blueberries, almonds, and a drizzle of honey	Tuna salad sandwich on whole-wheat bread with lettuce and tomato	Baked white fish with roasted asparagus and quinoa
8	Eggs (2) scrambled with tomatoes and feta cheese, with whole-wheat toast	Leftovers from dinner (baked fish)	Chicken breast stuffed with spinach and feta, served with sweet potatoes & roasted Brussels sprouts to taste
9	Greek yogurt with mixed berries and a sprinkle of hemp seeds	Lentil soup with whole-wheat bread and a side salad (arugula, pear, walnuts)	Vegetarian chili with kidney beans, corn, and avocado
10	Smoothie (banana, kale, almond milk, protein powder)	Leftovers from dinner (vegetarian chili)	Salmon cakes with roasted vegetables and a dill yogurt sauce

11	Oatmeal with banana slices and chopped pecans	Salad with chickpeas, cucumber, tomatoes, red onion, and a lemon-tahini dressing	Turkey meatballs with zucchini noodles and marinara sauce
12	Greek yogurt with mixed berries and a sprinkle of flax seeds	Leftovers from dinner (turkey meatballs)	Chicken stir-fry with broccoli, carrots, and brown rice
13	Eggs (2) sunny-side up with avocado toast	Tuna salad lettuce wraps with cucumber and carrot sticks	Baked cod with roasted cauliflower and quinoa
14	Smoothie (banana, spinach, almond milk, protein powder)	Leftovers from dinner (baked cod)	Celebrate completing the 14-day plan with a favorite meal that fits the guidelines!

Notes:

- **Portion Sizes:** Adjust portion sizes based on individual needs and activity levels.
- **Variety:** Feel free to swap out ingredients for similar options based on preference or availability.
- **Seasonings:** Use herbs, spices, and other healthy flavorings to enhance the taste of your meals.
- **Supplements:** Consider adding a high-quality probiotic and omega-3 supplement to your daily routine for additional gut and brain health support.

Additional Tips:

- **Listen to your body:** Eat when you're hungry, stop when you're full.

- **Stay hydrated:** You can shoot for 8 glasses of water every day.
- **Limit processed foods:** Avoid sugary drinks, refined grains, and fried foods.
- **Experiment:** You can unlock the power of experiment here by trying your hands on new recipes and ingredients to spice up your meals.
- **Be patient:** Healing takes time, and your diet is just one piece of the puzzle.

Important Note: This is a general guideline, and your needs might vary. And for all personalized demands and advice, it's advisable that you see a healthcare professional or registered dietitian.

Conclusion

The journey through trauma is undeniably challenging, but within the realm of somatic exercises lies a treasure trove of tools to aid healing and recovery.

"Somatic Exercises for Trauma" has taken you through effective techniques and exercises designed to bridge the gap between your mind and body, offering you pathways to reintegration, self-compassion, and profound transformation.

For pendulation, this technique teaches us the beauty of contrast, enabling our bodies to oscillate between tension and relaxation. In this dance of sensations, we learn to embrace the ebb and flow of emotions, gaining a deeper understanding and acceptance of ourselves. The practice encourages mindfulness, allowing us to track our moods and reconnect with the present moment, grounding us in the here and now.

This guide also stresses the need to nurture physical contact, through that we can create a sanctuary of safety within ourselves, providing a gentle embrace for our emotions and a beacon of light in moments of darkness. These exercises serve as gentle reminders that we are not alone on this journey; we have the power to soothe, comfort, and heal ourselves from within.

Another point dominant in this guide is that, by surrendering to instinctive motions and embracing free-flowing movements, we align ourselves with the natural cadences that resonate deep within our being. These practices encourage us to move intuitively, fostering a sense of harmony, balance, and interconnectedness with ourselves and the world around us.

Through therapeutic yoga postures, free dance, and targeted stretches, we release stored tension, clear stagnant energy, and cultivate a deeper sense of embodiment. These practices empower us to express, release, and rejuvenate, enabling us to feel more at home in our skin.

By engaging in expansive stretches, full-body shakes, and ancient practices like qigong and tai chi, we learn to cultivate and optimize our bioenergy circulation. These exercises serve as powerful tools for breaking through energetic blockages, dissipating chronic tension, and revitalizing our life force.

Lastly, exercises like *"When You Felt Most Like Yourself"* and *"Notice Your Current Physical Comfort"* encourage introspection and mindfulness. By reflecting on moments of authenticity and comfort, we gain insight into our emotional and physical states, fostering emotional regulation, nervous system regulation, and a greater sense of groundedness.

In conclusion, **"Somatic Exercises for Trauma & Anxiety"** is not just a guidebook but a companion on your healing journey. Each exercise is a stepping stone, guiding you towards self-discovery, self-compassion, and holistic well-being.

As you embrace these practices, remember that healing is a personal and ongoing process. Be patient with yourself, celebrate your progress, and trust in the innate wisdom of your body to guide you toward healing, resilience, and transformation. Your journey toward healing begins within, and somatic exercises are your roadmap to reclaiming your body, mind, and spirit.

CLAIM YOUR BONUSES HERE

Congratulations on walking this path with me. I'm excited to be part of your journey towards healing and transformation.

And I'm so grateful that you've chosen my book, "Somatic Exercises for Trauma and Anxiety," to guide you on your journey.

As a special thank you, I've put together **3 bonus resources** to help you deepen your practice and accelerate your healing. To access your bonuses, simply follow these easy steps:

1. Open your phone's camera and point it at the QR code below. Your camera should automatically recognize the code and show a link.

2. Tap the link, and it will take you to a special page leading you to your bonuses.

I'm excited to see how you use these additional tools to support your journey towards healing and well-being.

Remember, you are not alone. I am here to support you every step of the way.

References

Evans, A. T., & Hadler, N. M. (2006). Yoga improved function and reduced symptoms of chronic low-back pain more than a self-care book. ACP Journal Club. https://doi.org/10.7326/acpjc-2006-145-1-016

Osteopathic manual treatment and ultrasound therapy for chronic low back pain: A randomized controlled trial – Fingerprint — HSC. https://experts.unthsc.edu/en/publications/osteopathic-manual-treatment-and-ultrasound-therapy-for-chronic-l/fingerprints/

Body to Body Massage: A Tactile Ticket to Total Tranquility - Soho Asian Massage. https://www.sohoasianmassage.com/body-to-body-massage/body-to-body-massage-a-tactile-ticket-to-total-tranquility/

Printed in Great Britain
by Amazon

8c457faf-f80a-4189-8f64-d95e2aba908dR01